ALSO BY JANICE COX

Natural Beauty at Home

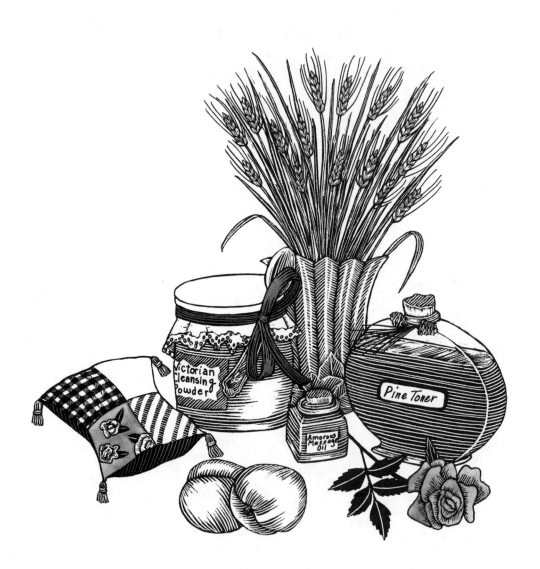

Natural Beauty for All Seasons

MORE THAN 250 SIMPLE RECIPES AND
GIFT-GIVING IDEAS FOR YEAR-ROUND BEAUTY

Janice Cox

Illustrated by Dorothy Reinhardt

An Owl Book
Henry Holt and Company
New York

Henry Holt and Company, Inc.
Publishers since 1866
115 West 18th Street
New York, New York 10011

Henry Holt® is a registered
trademark of Henry Holt and Company, Inc.

Published in Canada by Fitzhenry & Whiteside Ltd.,
195 Allstate Parkway, Markham, Ontario L3R 4T8.

Library of Congress Cataloging-in-Publication Data
Cox, Janice.
Natural beauty for all seasons: more than 250 simple recipes and gift-
giving ideas for year-round beauty / Janice Cox; illustrated by
Dorothy Reinhardt. — 1st ed.
          p.   cm.
"An owl book."
Includes index.
1. Beauty, Personal.   2. Skin — Care and hygiene.   3. Hair — Care
and hygiene.   4. Herbal cosmetics.   I. Title.
RA778.C755   1996   96-25025
646.7'2 — dc20   CIP

ISBN 0-8050-4655-0

Henry Holt books are available for special promotions and
premiums. For details contact: Director, Special Markets.

First Edition — 1996

DESIGNED BY LUCY ALBANESE

1   3   5   7   9   10   8   6   4   2

To my wonderful husband, Ray,
and my two precious daughters,
Lauren and Marie —
Your constant love and support
give my life true beauty!

Acknowledgments

I am extremely lucky to have good friends, a fabulous family, a super agent, the perfect editor, and a wonderful publisher—all were invaluable in creating this book.

To all of my friends and family: You are a constant source of inspiration and feedback.

To my agent, Laurie Harper: Thank you for your advice and friendship.

To my editor at Henry Holt and Company, Theresa Burns: Thank you again for your guidance. I love working with you through all of the seasons!

Special thank-yous to Raquel Jaramillo for another stunning cover design, Lucy Albanese for the overall book design, and Dorothy Reinhardt for her gorgeous artwork.

A final thank-you to everyone at Henry Holt and Company for your efforts in making this such a beautiful and special book.

We are all born with natural beauty; it is how we choose to use it that makes us unique. You are all beautiful!

Note

Contents

Autumn Skin and Hair Care *191*

Introduction

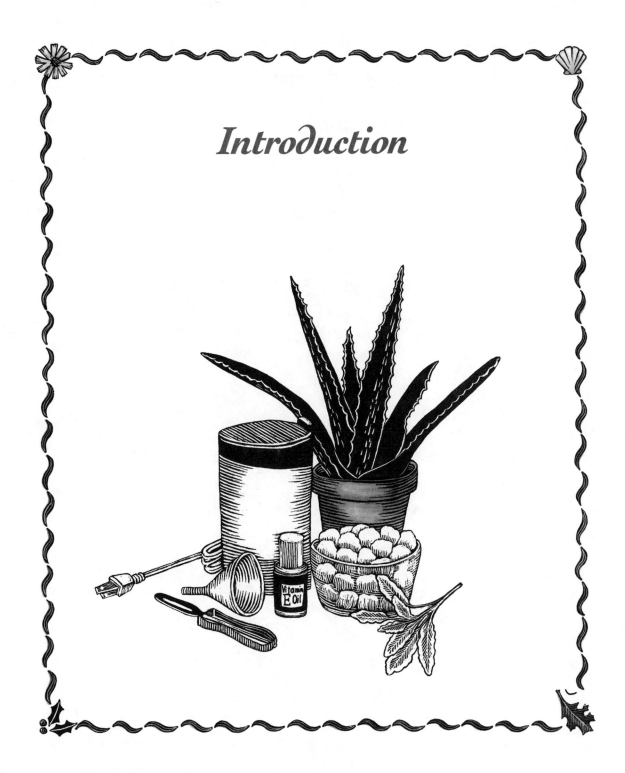

*M*y first book, *Natural Beauty at Home,* was a collection of favorite home beauty recipes and treatments, some of them handed down from three generations of my family. My grandmother just celebrated her ninety-first birthday. She is a beautiful woman who still enjoys her own "homemade" beauty treatments best.

You may be reading this book because you have found making your own cosmetic products to be a very satisfying experience and, like me, enjoy new recipes and ideas. If, on the other hand, this is a new area of interest for you, welcome!

I keep all the letters that I receive from friends and readers in a large basket next to my desk. Whenever I get a case of "writer's block" or need a friendly boost, I reread a sampling of the hundreds of wonderful and encouraging letters that were sent to me after I wrote *Natural Beauty at Home.* One theme that seems to run through them is how much *fun* everyone is having when making and sharing their own natural cosmetic products after using my recipes. I have always known these products and treatments could be entertaining and beneficial to your hair and skin, but hearing it from others always brings me joy!

In this book I present more than 250 brand-new, simple recipes and gift ideas for your body, bath, and hair. But this time I've organized the treatments by season, selecting the time of year when they are most effective and the ingredients are easiest to find. For instance, in the autumn, I tend to use apples, cranberries, nuts, and persimmons in my treatments. Spices, citrus fruits, and rich oils help keep me warm and looking my best in the winter. When the temperatures begin to rise, I turn to my garden for inspiration and use fresh flowers, fruits, vegetables, and herbs through the spring and summer months.

My routines and treatments also tend to change during the year. My skin and hair are much drier during the cold winter months, so I like to use more oil-rich products and never go to bed without using a night cream. Winter products featured here include recipes for lip balms, mustard baths, scented massage oils, and hair conditioners. In the warmer months I tend to cleanse my hair and skin more often and enjoy lighter, "cooler" products. Garden colognes, skin toners, and facial masks using fresh fruits are a few of the many spring and summer products I like to use. Please note that this arrangement of recipes by season is merely a guideline. If there is a product that you enjoy using, there's no reason you can't use it whenever you want!

I have also given more attention in this book to the subject of gift-giving — a favorite topic of my readers. I have always loved making my own presents and have encouraged my two daughters to do the same. It is hard to put into words the feeling when a grateful recipient says, "I can't believe you made this!" We have many gift-giving holidays and special occasions, including Mother's Day, Father's Day, graduations, birthdays, births, and weddings. Included in many of these recipes are ideas and packaging tips. Use them as a starting point to get your creative juices flowing.

I give credit to my parents for allowing me to experiment and practice my recipes at a very young age. My laboratory was the family bathroom. I would spend hours locked away with old recipes, magazine clippings, and my chemistry textbooks. My parents were very tolerant of my beauty interest and only occasionally would my father express surprise when I emerged with an egg facial or my hair covered in henna paste. I even recruited my sister, Mariann, to be a co-manager of our own exclusive, after-school beauty salon.

I am now married to a wonderful man, and we have two natural beauties. I still spend hours trying out new beauty treatments, recipes, and cosmetic formulas. I love it when I overhear my husband admitting to his friends that a facial mask "really does feel great"!

In addition to the satisfaction I receive from making my own cosmetic products, the cost savings are also attractive. When you realize what you have been spending on commercial products (a majority of the price is based on packaging and advertising, not the cost of the actual ingredients), you will be amazed and delighted at the cost of home treatments. I have seen gorgeous bottles of colored bath salts for up to $50 in department stores; you can create your own very similar products for under $2!

The recipes in this book are easy to follow and use common ingredients that can be found in your local supermarket or natural food store. The recipes call for modern kitchen equipment such as a saucepan, measuring cups, and a blender—nothing exotic. Many of the procedures involve simply mixing together a few ingredients in the right proportions. None of the recipes requires any more skill than boiling water and being able to follow directions.

Each year we have the opportunity to live four seasons of beauty and

---

TEN STEPS TO NATURAL BEAUTY

1. Get plenty of rest.

2. Exercise regularly.

3. Eat a balanced diet.

4. Take breaks to boost your energy. Meditate, relax, or walk.

5. Keep your skin and hair clean and full of moisture.

6. Use sun protection.

7. Brush and floss your teeth regularly.

8. Drink plenty of water—at least eight glasses a day.

9. Give yourself a monthly total body treatment (head to toe).

10. Use natural beauty products.

health, and you can use the recipes, gift ideas, and treatments in this book to look and feel terrific in all of them. Most important, you'll have fun. And keep those letters of inspiration coming my way!

A WORD ABOUT THE RECIPES

The recipes in this book do not contain any artificial colors or fragrance, and many can be made fragrance-free. Different scents are often suggested, but these are always optional ingredients. The color and scent of these products are derived from their own natural ingredients. These look and smell wonderful on their own as nature intended!

Preservatives are not needed for most of these recipes because certain ingredients act as natural preservatives—vitamin E, vitamin C, and tincture of benzoin, for example—or the amount the recipe yields is enough for one application. If you choose not to use a preservative that has been suggested, that product may need refrigeration.

If you are sensitive to a known ingredient—say, olive oil—either find a suitable substitution, such as almond oil, or choose a different recipe. You should know that you can be as sensitive to natural beauty products as to commercial products. If you have a known food allergy, such as tomatoes, chances are you will also be allergic to a cosmetic product that contains tomatoes even though you're not ingesting it. Care should always be taken when using a new product or treatment. Always spot-test it first: Apply a small amount to the skin on the inside of your arm and wait twenty-four hours. If there is no reaction, it is probably safe to proceed with the treatment. If you have extremely sensitive skin or have a long list of allergies, it is always best to consult a dermatologist or physician before using any new product or treatment. Remember, you are the manufacturer of these cosmetic products, and quality control is therefore *your* responsibility. And be sure to always work with clean equipment and pure ingredients.

The following is a list of basic care and storage guidelines to ensure a long and healthy shelf life for your homemade cosmetic products:

1. Always store your products in the cleanest of jars and bottles.

2. Try to keep your fingers out of the container as much as possible. Always wash your hands before handling cosmetics. Remember that each time you dip your fingers into the containers, foreign germs and materials are introduced. Try to use cotton balls, cotton swabs, or a small spatula when possible, or *pour* your products onto clean hands.

3. Store your products in a cool, dark, dry place. Heat and light can sometimes alter their composition.

4. If the ingredients in the product separate, don't worry. Simply stir the mixture thoroughly or recombine using a hand mixer or blender.

5. If something smells bad or changes color, it probably is best to throw it out. Once a product has gone bad, there is no way to recover it. It's best to make a new batch.

NATURAL BEAUTY TOOLS AND EQUIPMENT

Below is a list of tools you will need for making the cosmetics and beauty treatments in this book. Many are common kitchen items that you already own. You will probably not need all the items listed; for example, a blender, an electric mixer, or a spoon can be used for stirring. Remember to keep your equipment clean; you don't want to introduce any foreign ingredients into your cosmetic products.

Grater: I like to use a standard handheld metal cheese grater for beeswax, soap, and vegetables.

Vegetable peeler: For peeling vegetables and grating beeswax and soap. I prefer to use a vegetable peeler for grating beeswax and cocoa butter since it is faster and easier to clean.

Citrus peeler and zester: For removing the peel or "zest" (colored part of the peel) of citrus fruits. It's not essential, but it's a fun gadget to use. You can do just as well with a sharp paring knife.

Measuring cups and spoons: A must for measuring ingredients correctly.

Glass ovenproof measuring cups with pouring spouts: I use these for everything. They can be put in a hot-water bath, the microwave, and the refrigerator. Glass will not react with any of your cosmetic ingredients and is easy to clean.

Stirring rod: I use a chopstick for a stirring rod. It isn't essential, but it makes stirring small amounts easy. It also makes me feel like more of a chemist.

Pans: Steel and enamel pans work best. Aluminum and iron sometimes react with ingredients, especially when making soap.

Microwave: Not entirely necessary, but it really speeds things up, especially heating and melting times.

Blender and/or food processor: Perfect for really mixing up creams and lotions. You can mix pretty well by hand, but a blender makes the task so much easier and faster. Make sure your blender is dishwasher-safe to cut down on cleaning time.

Hand mixer or electric whisk: Speeds up mixing of creams and lotions as a blender does, but because it is handheld, you have a little more direct control.

Coffee grinder: For grinding peels and herbs. Make sure you clean it well after each use or your coffee may taste a bit funny! Spice grinders and small food processors also work well.

Funnel: For bottling your products and filtering solutions.

Coffee filters, cheesecloth, paper towels: All can be used as filtering material to be placed inside funnels and strainers when solutions and mixtures are to be poured through.

Knives: For cutting and chopping.

Glass and ceramic bowls: For mixing, heating in the microwave, and storing products.

WEIGHTS AND MEASURES

3 teaspoons = 1 tablespoon
4 tablespoons = ¼ cup
8 tablespoons = ½ cup
12 tablespoons = ¾ cup
16 tablespoons = 1 cup
1 cup = 8 ounces
1 cup = ½ pint
2 cups = 1 pint
4 cups = 1 quart
4 quarts = 1 gallon
juice of 1 lemon = about 3 tablespoons
juice of 1 orange = about ⅓ cup

METRIC EQUIVALENTS

1 ounce = 28.35 grams
1 gram = 0.035 ounce
1 quart = 0.946 liter
1 liter = 1.06 quarts

Eyedropper: For adding scents and natural preservatives.

Strainer: For straining solutions and mixtures.

Old muffin tins, loaf pans, and cookie cutters: Used as molds when making soap.

Stove top, warming plate, or electric skillet: You will need heat to melt ingredients in some of the recipes. If you do not have a stove available, you can use an electric skillet with one to two inches of water to create a water bath.

Assorted jars, bottles, bowls, and spray bottles: For storing and applying your cosmetics. These containers can be found in a variety of places: grocery stores, drugstores, department stores, and stores specializing in cooking equipment. Put your recycling creativity to use: Before throwing out an old jar, bottle, or container, think of how it could be reused for your own cosmetics products. Plastic honey bears and "sport drink" squeeze bottles are great for lotions, shampoos, and liquid soaps. Wine and liquor bottles are perfect for scented oils and bath mixtures. Even your old commercial cosmetic containers can be used to hold your new homemade versions.

CARING FOR YOUR BEAUTY TOOLS

The combs, brushes, and other tools you use to keep your skin and hair looking their best also need care. Keeping them clean will not only make them last longer but will keep harmful bacteria from developing and being passed onto your skin and hair.

Brushes and combs should be washed regularly. Remove any loose hair. Fill a sink or large bucket with warm water and add 1 tablespoon of baking soda and ⅛ teaspoon of bleach or other antiseptic. Soak brushes and combs for 15 to 20 minutes, then rinse well and allow to air-dry completely. Wooden combs and brushes should not be washed but brushed clean and protected with a light coating of oil.

Manicure tools and nail clippers should be washed after each use in hot water and a mild detergent. Soak scissors in alcohol and allow them to air-dry completely. Store your tools by wrapping them in a clean, dry towel.

Razors should also be cleaned after each use and allowed to dry out completely. The worst place to store your razor is in the shower because the warm moist air speeds up bacteria growth. Soak your razor once a week in alcohol and allow it to air-dry. Change razor blades regularly.

Loofah sponges should be cleaned monthly by soaking them in a 10 percent bleach solution and allowed to air-dry thoroughly. If used regularly, they should be discarded every couple of months.

Cosmetic tools such as sponge applicators, facial brushes, and tweezers should also be washed in a mild detergent and left to air-dry completely.

Toothbrushes should also air-dry completely between uses and should be disinfected every couple of weeks. If the bristles look worn or bent, get a new brush. In any case, they should be replaced every three months.

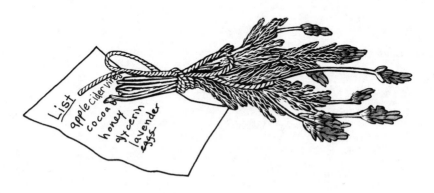

A Seasonal
Shopping Guide

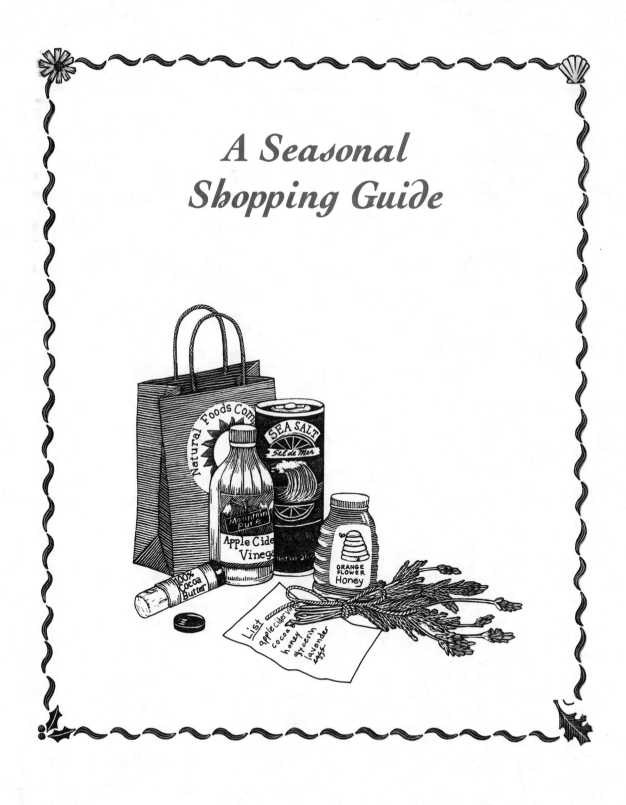

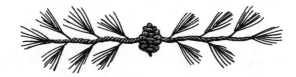

New and different natural ingredients appear with each change of season—for example, spring flowers, summer herbs, autumn grains, and winter citrus fruits—and, of course, beauty basics such as eggs, milk, salt, and natural oils are available year-round. But some of the fresh ingredients are available only during certain growing seasons. Where I live, fresh figs, which are wonderful natural skin exfoliators, are available only in the fall.

We are lucky to live in a world in which air transportation has extended the growing seasons and expanded the local produce offerings. I was pleasantly surprised this past summer to find a wide selection of tropical fruits grown in other countries at my local produce stand, and many summer-only fruits, such as strawberries, are now available year-round. You will, however, pay more for out-of-season crops. I prefer to use what is available fresh at the market, changing my cosmetic ingredients and routines with each new season. I also think my skin and hair benefit from this seasonal approach to beauty.

I have put together a list of the primary natural ingredients used throughout this book, organized by season. You are already familiar with many of them because they are common household staples, but others will be exciting new discoveries. This is not, of course, a comprehensive list. You will also find information about ingredients in the introductions to individual recipes and treatments.

During the cold, crisp winter months, fresh produce is at a minimum at my grocery store, but not to worry! During this time of year I turn to my pantry shelves for inspiration and beauty ingredients, and enjoy using dried ingredients, dairy products, and fragrant spices in my winter recipes. One of my all-time-favorite winter ingredients is pure maple syrup. It's a natural humectant, so it keeps my skin soft and radiant, and does wonders for dry winter hair. Here are a few more of my favorite winter ingredients:

Baking soda: Available year-round at your local grocery store. Baking soda is a gentle, alkaline, white powder that neutralizes acids. It has a multitude of beauty uses: as a deodorant, a bath powder, an addition to dusting powder, and as a simple tooth whitener. (Lately I've even been using it as a hair rinse!) Mixed with water it helps remove residues from hairstyling products and makes my hair really clean and shiny.

Beans: Dried beans are rich in protein, potassium, and iron. Finely ground into a powder, they make a terrific cleanser for the face and body. Simply mix the ground beans together with a bit of water or your favorite skin cleanser and massage into damp skin. Red kidney, pink azuki, lima beans, and black beans are all good skin conditioners to try. Dried beans are easily found at your local supermarket.

Beer: Beer is a classic hair rinse and setting lotion that my mother used all the time when she was young. The flatter the beer—meaning the less carbonation in it—the better. The sugar and protein in beer work to thicken the hair. I like to spray my hair with flat beer before setting it on electric rollers. I have also found the more inexpensive beers work the best when used in my beauty recipes!

Cherimoya: This tropical fruit grown in Peru is available in many markets only in the winter months. It is sometimes referred to as the "custard fruit" because of its creamy white interior that tastes like a mild fruit custard.

Cherimoyas are moisturizing and soothing to dry skin—the fresh fruit pulp makes a wonderful facial treatment.

Citrus fruits: I was raised in a family of orange growers. Both of my grandfathers and my father grew oranges in Southern California. This is probably why citrus fruits are my favorite beauty ingredients. I still love to float whole oranges in my bath, use lemon juice as a rinse when my hair is tired and dull, and clean my whole body with ground citrus peels. Lemons, oranges, tangerines, and limes all make good winter ingredients for cosmetics because of their citric acid content. Citric acid kills bacteria on the skin, and the fresh scent is a known energizer. Citrus fruits are also some of the few "fresh" fruits available during the winter months.

Cocoa butter: Cocoa butter, which comes from the seeds of the cacao plant, is a creamy, fatty wax that is solid at room temperature. Chocolate lovers will enjoy cocoa butter's mild chocolate scent. It is an excellent skin softener and can be used alone or mixed with other ingredients. Hollywood beauty legend Mae West often used pure cocoa butter to keep her skin soft and smooth.

Dairy products: Milk, cream, yogurt, and sour cream are all high in protein, calcium, and vitamins, and make soothing cleansers. They also contain lactose, an alpha hydroxy acid that gently sloughs off dead cells, leaving your skin soft and smooth. Milk baths were made popular by the Egyptian Queen Cleopatra, who was known for her incomparable beauty. It is important to rinse well after using dairy products because the milk will spoil if left on your skin.

Maple syrup: Maple syrup is made from boiling the sap of the sugar maple tree and is a natural humectant, a material that holds in moisture. It can be used as a facial mask, as a hair conditioner, and in lots of bath treatments. Pure maple syrup can be found at your local supermarket. Look for syrup marked 100 percent pure maple syrup for the best results.

Spices: Cinnamon, cloves, anise, nutmeg, black pepper, and ginger, to name just a few, are all wonderful ingredients in natural beauty products. These aromatic dried seeds, bark, and flower buds can be used in massage oils and fragrance products. They are also very useful in warming the body on a cold winter day. Try a bit of clove or cinnamon oil massaged into your feet and hands to warm and relax them. Spices can add drama to your tresses when used as a hair rinse or added to henna paste. Sold in bulk or individual packages, they are easily found in any market or grocery store.

Tea tree oil: The leaves from the Australian tea tree (*Melaleuca alternifolia*) produce an oil that has powerful antibacterial and antiviral qualities. It is easily absorbed by the skin. In Australia the aborigines have been using this essential oil for centuries as a cure for a variety of ailments. Tea tree oil can now be purchased in any natural food store.

SPRING BEAUTY INGREDIENTS

After several months of cold weather and colorless scenery, the world suddenly becomes fragrant and green in spring! Even if you live in a desert climate, you will notice more green in the landscape. Fresh flowers, herbs, and more fresh produce such as rhubarb, lettuce, and carrots can be found in the grocery store. I welcome the occasional spring shower because it promotes one of the most beautiful aspects of spring: the growth of plants and flowers. I find myself looking skyward and letting the rainwater gently cover my face, adding moisture to my skin. Here is a list of my favorite spring ingredients:

Carrots: Carrots are rich in vitamin A, which is often called the beauty vitamin because it is essential for clear skin and shiny hair. Grated carrots used as a facial mask can hydrate the skin and help clear away dead cells. If you are having trouble with skin blemishes, washing your face with carrot juice is a good cure. Carrot oil, made from carrot seeds, is a light yellow essential oil that can be added to creams and lotions. It is available at natural food stores.

Eggs: Available year-round, eggs are associated with the season of spring because they are a symbol of rebirth and new beginnings. Eggs are rich in protein and make good skin and hair conditioners. Egg yolks are rich in lecithin, a natural emollient. Egg whites are naturally astringent, which means they help shrink or tighten your skin's pores. A gentle shampoo can be made by simply using a raw egg to clean your hair. Rinse well with cool water (hot water may cook the egg). Because eggs are inexpensive and easy to find, they are one of the most popular at-home beauty ingredients.

Essential oils: Essential oils are highly concentrated aromatic extracts of different plants (usually a single plant). They come in a variety of scents. Essential oils are pure and intense, and their fragrance will last a very long time. Add a few drops to your favorite body lotion, massage oil, or bathwater. I purchase these fragrant oils at health food stores or aromatherapy shops. (Aromatherapy is the practice of using scents to create or change your mood or mental state. It works through the sense of smell, which affects how we eat, our sexual drive, and our behavior in general.) When used in massage therapy, essential oils are usually added to a carrier oil such as almond or sesame oil.

Flowers: Nothing says spring to me like fresh flowers! Some of my favorites to use in cosmetics are lavender, lilac, rose, primrose, and pansy. You can purchase flowers from organic growers (make sure no pesticides are used on the flowers) or grow your own. Flowers that have wilted or turned a bit brown are still usable for cosmetics.

Flowers have been used in cosmetics for ages, often for symbolic reasons (for instance, lavender is believed to bring good luck to women). A flower's physical properties are also important. Roses, for example, are naturally astringent and help cleanse the skin, removing surface dirt and oils.

Lanolin: Lanolin is found in the oil glands of sheep and is more like a wax than an oil or fat. It absorbs and holds water next to the skin. It is available in two forms: anhydrous (without added water) and hydrous (with added water). Anhydrous lanolin is a thick golden liquid and is usually found at natural food stores. Lanolin creams can also be found in the baby section of the grocery store.

Lettuce: A crisp lettuce leaf can be rubbed directly on the skin to help combat oiliness. This is especially good for those with oily skin. A solution made from boiling fresh lettuce with water, when added to the bath, has been shown to promote sleep because it is high in sulfur, silicon, and phosphorous. Lettuce juice is also soothing to sunburned skin.

Orange flower water: Orange flower water is a fragrant water made from the blossoms of the bitter orange tree. The oil from this flower is called *neroli,* and its scent is believed to reduce stress and induce sleep. This fragrant water makes a gentle skin freshener. I keep a small spray bottle in my purse to use when I feel rundown at the end of a day or to pick me up when I'm traveling. You can find it in liquor stores in the mixer section and in many health food stores.

Rosewater: Another fragrant water, this time made from distilling fresh rose petals with water. Rose petals are naturally astringent. You can easily make your own rosewater by gently heating fresh rose petals in some distilled water and letting the mixture cool. I sometimes find rosewater at the liquor store (it's used in some specialty drinks). It is also sold at many pharmacies and health food stores.

Whey: Whey is a popular Scandinavian beauty secret. A by-product of cheese-making, it is rich in protein and can be used as an emollient in beauty recipes in place of dairy ingredients. I find powdered whey at my grocery store in the flour section.

SUMMER BEAUTY INGREDIENTS

During the summer months, fresh vegetables, fruits, flowers, and herbs are available in abundance. This is the time of year when the garden is in full bloom and farmer's markets are full of fresh produce. I also love to visit the beach and walk barefoot in the sand. On my walks I collect ingredients from the sea. Fresh kelp and seaweed, which bloom and grow in the ocean, are easy to find as they wash up on the shore. To cleanse my skin and hair I also love to use many of the exotic tropical fruits, such as papayas, pineapples, and kiwi fruits, which are so much easier to find in the summer. Here is the list of my favorite summer ingredients:

Aloe vera gel: Aloe vera plants are easy to grow and make a wonderful addition to your indoor plant collection. The leaves from the aloe vera plant contain a clear jellylike sap that promotes healing and cools and soothes the skin. It is naturally astringent, so you may want to mix a little with some vegetable oil if you have dry skin. Plain aloe vera gel makes a wonderful setting lotion for the hair and a great treatment for sunburn.

Avocado: Avocados are rich in natural oil, protein, and vitamins A and B. They make an excellent moisturizer for dry skin and hair. I like to use a mashed avocado in my hair once a week as a deep conditioner. Pale green avocado oil is available in many grocery and natural food stores today and makes a wonderful addition to creams and lotions. I even use avocado stones (pits) to make my body scrubs. Simply dry them out and finely grind them in a coffee grinder or food processor. For a triple avocado body scrub, mash half an avocado and mix with 1 tablespoon of avocado oil and 2 tablespoons of ground avocado stone.

Berries: Raspberries, blackberries, huckleberries, blueberries, and boysenberries—fresh summer berries are something I look forward to all year long. These jewel-colored delicacies will give your skin a rosy glow when used as a facial mask. The leaves of the raspberry and blackberry bush can be made into a strong tea and used in the bath or as a hair rinse. Crush a few red berries and add them to your favorite lip gloss recipe for a pretty, transparent tint.

Calendula: These sunny yellow-orange flowers are also known as "pot marigolds." The flower heads and petals can be used fresh or dried. Calendula is soothing to rough, dry skin. They are a natural antiseptic. You may purchase dried flower petals at many natural food stores or grow your own for a burst of color in your backyard.

Coconut: Coconut milk and coconut oil are both rich in natural emollients and oils. Coconut milk is easy to make from fresh coconuts and is an excellent addition to hair conditioners and body lotions. Coconut oil, which is a white solid oil at room temperature, preserves the skin and hair by providing a protective layer that locks in natural moisture. I like to rub a bit of coconut oil into my skin after showering.

Corn oil, corn milk, cornmeal, cornstarch: Many corn products are popular beauty ingredients. Corn oil and corn milk are soothing to dry skin because they are both rich emollients. Cornstarch has become a popular replacement for talcum powder and is a key ingredient in many natural dusting powders. It can also be used as a thickening agent in creams and lotions. Cornmeal makes a good all-purpose skin scrub. I like blue cornmeal because of its unique color.

Cucumbers: Women have been placing sliced cucumbers over their tired eyes for years. This simple and effective treatment cools and refreshes, and reduces eye puffiness. Fresh cucumber juice is also a mild astringent, perfect for cleansing delicate skin or soothing a bad sunburn. Cucumber juice is fragile and will not keep for long. Always store all products that contain fresh cucumber juice in the refrigerator to increase their shelf life.

Herbs: This is the season for growing and harvesting fresh herbs to use now and all year long. My personal favorites include chamomile, mint, lavender, sage, and basil. Besides the grocery store, herbs can also be found in abundant supply at roadside stands and farmer's markets. I like to make small, fresh herb wreaths to keep in my bathroom—I pick a few leaves or flowers and add them to my bathwater, whenever I feel like it.

Honey and beeswax: Busy summer bees produce two ingredients that can be used year-round: honey and beeswax. I keep a sharp eye out for beekeepers at farmer's markets because they are an excellent and cost-effective source of beeswax. This golden wax is secreted from the underside of the bees when they make the honeycomb. No synthetic product has yet to be developed that can boast the same properties. It is the key ingredient in many creams, lotions, and lip products. Honey is one of the best-known humectants and has a very high potassium content, which makes it almost impossible for bacteria to survive in it. My favorite way to use honey is to add it to bathwater. Just a small amount will make your skin feel like silk.

Roses: Not only are roses beautiful to look at, but they have also been an important ingredient in cosmetic products for centuries. Galen, the Greek physician from the second century, used rosewater and rose oil in many of his cosmetic formulas. Roses are naturally astringent and cleansing. Their heady scent never fails to summon feelings of romance and passion. I like to pick my roses in the early morning just after the dew has dried. I then lay the petals in a shallow basket to air-dry for later use.

Salt (sea salt, Epsom salts, table salt [sodium chloride]): Bath salts soothe tired muscles and soften the skin. They are highly soluble and do not leave any residue behind. Salt also softens hard water and can therefore prevent these deposits from forming in the tub. Adding salt to your bath also helps keep the water temperature warmer longer. Salt in a variety of forms is easily found at the grocery store. Epsom salts (magnesium sulfate) is usually in the health care section.

Seaweed: Sea plants are good for dry skin because they contain a large amount of iodine and protein. Seaweed can be added to bathwater, creams, and lotions. Some seaweed, such as Irish moss, can be used to thicken hair gels and creams. For a quick and easy thalassotherapy, or sea water therapy treatment, add a tablespoon or two of dried seaweed to a warm bath and create your own mini-ocean. Natural food stores and Asian markets are a good source for dried seaweed.

Sunflower oil and seeds: Sunflowers have become a welcome symbol of summer for my family. My daughters love to plant these giant flowers in our yard each year (sometimes in surprise locations). Sunflower oil is rich in vitamin E and makes a good skin lotion or massage oil. Sunflower seeds (shelled, of course) make a good all-over body scrub. Mix together with a bit of sunflower oil or lotion. Sunflower oil and seeds are easily found at the grocery store.

Tropical fruits (pineapple, papaya, banana, mango): Warmer weather brings a colorful supply of tropical fruits to local markets. I was pleased to see the large tropical papaws that come from Australia at my local market this year, along with kiwis, pineapples, and coconuts. They can be used to remove dead skin (pineapple and papaya), moisturize (banana and coconut), and refresh (mango and kiwi).

Water: Water is the major component of all living things and the most common ingredient in cosmetics today. The best beauty treatment of all is to drink at least eight glasses of water a day (a little more on hot summer days). One of the most overlooked causes of fatigue may be the easiest to cure. Dehydration can lead to headaches, irritability, and a general rundown feeling. Even your hair and skin will look dull and lifeless without the proper amount of water in your system. So, drink up!

AUTUMN BEAUTY INGREDIENTS

During the autumn months, many of the natural beauty ingredients I choose to use come from fields and trees and are rich in texture and color. They include fresh grains, nuts, and fall fruits such as pears, apples, and persimmons. Root vegetables are also collected this time of year; fresh potatoes, parsnips, and yams are all in ample supply. Living in Oregon, I am lucky to have fresh nuts such as hazelnuts and walnuts available during this season. Here is the list of my favorite autumn ingredients:

Apples: Some of the oldest folk remedies include apples. They have been known for centuries for their skin-healing power. Apple juice makes a breath-sweetening mouth rinse and can also be used in skin toners and in the bath. The juice contains malic acid, which acts as an antioxidant in cosmetic recipes, and amylase, which is an exfoliating enzyme useful in removing dead skin cells and surface dirt. Apple juice can even be used as a hair rinse to control dandruff! The seeds are mildly poisonous and should not be used.

Artichokes: An excellent skin and hair conditioner, artichokes contain potassium and vitamin A. I like to mash freshly steamed artichoke hearts with a bit of wheat germ oil and a teaspoon of apple cider vinegar and apply it to my hair thirty minutes before shampooing. They can be found especially during the fall in any grocery store.

Cranberries: These bright berries make an excellent skin tonic. They boost your circulation and give your face a healthy glow. Fresh cranberries can be found in the grocery store this time of year and freeze well for use all year long. You can tell if your berries are fresh if they bounce when dropped on the counter or floor. The majority of cranberries are grown in bogs in New England, but due to their increasing popularity, several new bogs have been planted in many other parts of the country.

Figs: Fresh figs are wonderful skin cleansers and mild exfoliators. Like pineapple and papaya, they contain an active natural enzyme that helps remove dead cells from the skin's surface. They are extremely perishable and should be used as quickly as possible. I see fresh figs in the market from late summer through the early months of fall. I use them as a body scrub in the shower; their soft flesh and tiny seeds polish my skin. If fresh figs are hard to find, simply use dried ones. Soak them in water for twenty minutes before using in recipes.

Grains: Barley, wheat, and oats, all whole grains, are valuable sources of protein, vitamin E, and the B vitamins. Finely ground, they make an excellent cleanser that can be used in place of soap. Added to your bathwater, they create a soothing soak perfect for all skin types. Oatmeal baths are a popular cure for dry, sensitive skin. You can make small bath bags to tie under your water tap by stitching together two squares of cheesecloth and filling them with fresh grains.

Nuts: Almonds, walnuts, and hazelnuts are all harvested in the fall and are rich in natural oils. The expressed oils can be found in the cooking oil section of your local grocery store or gourmet food shop, year-round. Finely ground nuts make excellent face and body scrubs.

Potatoes: Rich in vitamin C, these root vegetables are wonderful skin soothers and are an effective remedy for dry, flaky skin. Simply rub a slice of raw potato over your skin, then rinse. Potato slices also help reduce puffiness when placed over tired eyes. I like to use russet potatoes, but all types work well. Make sure to remove the outer peel first because it may discolor your skin slightly.

Rose hips: Rose hips are the fully ripened orange-red fruits, about the size of a cherry, just below the rose flower. They are picked in the late fall, just before the frost destroys them. All roses have "hips," but only certain species of the rose have a fruit suitable for eating. Rosa Rugosa is the most common fruit-bearing variety in the United States. Dried and powdered rose hips can be found at your local natural food store. Rose hips are rich in vitamin C and make wonderful skin toners and facial masks.

Vinegar: When fruit juice ferments, it turns into vinegar, known for its high acid content and sharp odor. In cosmetics, vinegar is used to remove alkaline residues from soap products and helps restore our body's own natural acid level. You should never use straight vinegar on your skin; always dilute it with water (try one part vinegar to eight parts water). My favorite way to use scented vinegars is in the bath; they remove dry flaky skin and leave my whole body aglow.

Witch hazel: Hamamelis virginiana, or witch hazel, is a plant that flowers in late autumn. Its bark and leaves can be made into a wonderful skin freshener, local anesthetic, and astringent. It's been a staple of medicine chests for at least three hundred years. My grandmother soothes her tired eyes by soaking two cotton pads in witch hazel and putting them on her lids while she rests for ten minutes. Witch hazel can be found at any pharmacy and in the health care section of the grocery store.

The Art of
Natural Gift-Giving

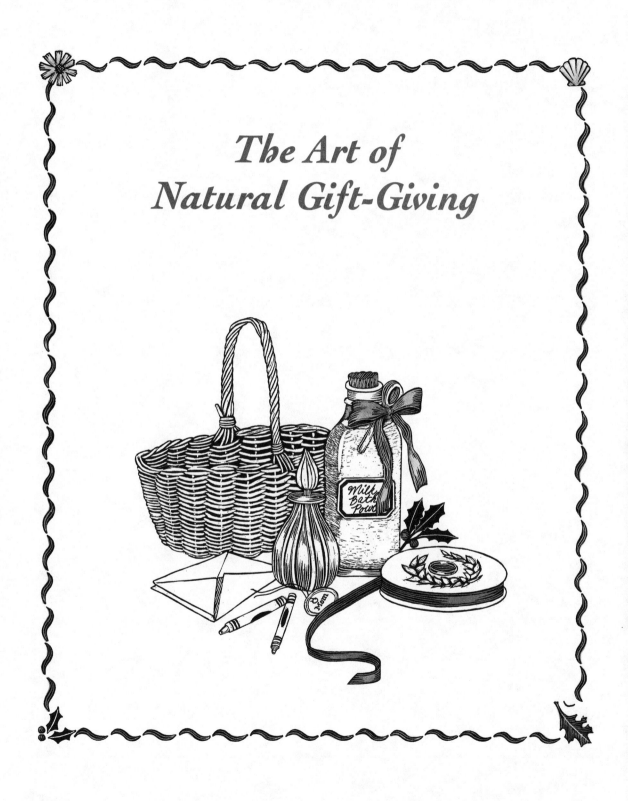

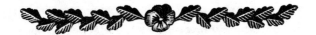

I have three basic rules in gift-giving:

- Give what you would like to receive.
- Personalize your gift.
- Be creative!

Whenever I cannot think of what to get someone for a gift, I say to myself, "What would I like if I were that person?" For a friend who is an avid road runner I came up with a wonderful assortment of beauty products that would fit a very active person. An energizing toner, soothing massage oil, and scented shower gel went into a new hip pack along with a brightly colored water bottle and a new runner's hat to protect her hair. For another friend who just had a baby, I thought back to my own first days of motherhood and put together a beautiful basket filled with pampering bath products that I would have loved to receive! I even included a few soothing products, such as some lavender oil for her new daughter.

Personalizing your gifts makes them even more unique. This can be done by using favorite colors or scents. My grandmother is crazy about anything blue and loves cats. I once saw some bath towels with white cat faces on them and had to get them for her. Packaged together with some new blue bath salts, it was the perfect present. You can also personalize your gifts by decorating the packages with names, poems, artwork, and favorite quotes. Plain glass bottles become a work of art when decorated with colorful paint (check with your local craft or hobby shop for special glass paint). Make special envelopes to hold dry products such as powders, bath products, or clay for facial masks. Include a small note inside each envelope.

Be creative. Don't be afraid to try something new or give something a bit unusual. A champagne bucket filled with massage oils, scented candles, and romantic music could be the start of an evening to remember. A large tote bag filled with travel essentials is the perfect bon voyage gift for a jet-setting friend. Remember, everyone loves to be surprised and pampered. I have given baskets to couples, grandmothers, young brides, executives, and baby-sitters—and have received warm hugs from all.

The best gifts are those that are truly from the heart. Give of yourself, and you will receive much more than can be expressed by mere words. It is one of the greatest joys in this world, and something we should all have a chance to experience!

PACKAGING YOUR PRODUCTS

Advertisers and manufacturers everywhere know that it's hard for anyone to resist an inviting package. I have even been known to buy a product for its packaging alone. It's easy to create beautiful and professional-looking designs for your own products using simple household, craft, and office supplies.

Bottles and jars—especially old, uncommon ones—when filled with bath and beauty products make wonderful presents. Imagine an old milk bottle filled with a fragrant powdered milk bath or an antique perfume bottle containing my Summer Garden Cologne (see page 179). I am always on the lookout for unusual containers at garage sales and antique shops. Import stores and bath shops carry a wide range of newer jars and bottles, and I have also found great ones in restaurant supply shops, medical supply houses, kitchen stores, and gardening centers. Before placing any empty glass container into the recycling bin, always consider how it might be used for your natural beauty products. With their labels removed and a new cork top or painted lid, those salad dressing and jelly jars can be transformed into works of art! For products used in the shower or by children, use plastic containers instead of glass, since they don't break if dropped on tile floors.

Bottles and jars should be absolutely clean and dry before adding any substance to them. The simplest way to remove labels is with a good soaking in warm soapy water. I usually fill a plastic bucket and let the jars and bottles soak overnight. Really stubborn labels can be removed using a bit of vegetable oil, which loosens up the glue. Simply rub a bit all over the label; you may need to "score" or scrape the label with a sharp knife. Use very hot water and always let the containers air-dry completely. Moisture can ruin some products, such as powders and oils. If you want to speed up the drying process, pour a small amount of alcohol such as vodka into the container, swirl it around, then pour out. The alcohol will displace all the water as it evaporates and reduce the overall drying time.

Paint can be removed from the bottles using inexpensive hair spray or alcohol; you may also have to scrub a bit with fine steel wool. You can spray-paint jar lids. They even have colors now that resemble rock surfaces. Or cover the lids with bits of wrapping paper or fabric.

Special marking pens, available at many craft and art supply stores, can be used on glass, and stickers that resemble etched glass designs can be placed on your containers. Be creative!

New stoppers and corks can be purchased at hardware stores or stores that sell wine-making equipment. (Look in your yellow pages under wine-making supplies.) These are also a good source for bottles. Use a small rubber mallet to gently tap the corks into your bottles. A wax seal on top of your homemade products helps keep air and dirt out and gives them a more professional look. Create your own using kitchen paraffin, old candles, beeswax, and crayons. Melt beeswax, kitchen paraffin (used for jams and jellies), or candles in a double boiler or microwave container. Dip the bottle into the melted wax or brush the wax onto the lid. Let each layer harden briefly. Apply several layers until the package has the look you desire. For colored wax, I use small bits of my daughters' broken crayons. Add the crayons to the melted wax and stir slowly. Some people like to wrap a ribbon over the bottle top with the ends hanging down before dipping it in the wax. This makes removing the wax easier—simply pull on the loose ribbon ends, and the wax seal lifts right off. Today the wine industry is changing to "naked" corks. Bottles are simply corked and a dot of beeswax is put in place to create a seal. Try this look for sealing bath oils and lotions; the beeswax has a warm honey color.

Always label your products. This is especially important when giving them as gifts. Be sure to list all the ingredients, adding any instructions for use, such as: "Pour ½ cup into the bath under running water." I like to collect old and unusual labels. These can be reproduced easily using a copy machine (for color, use a color copier). At your local library you may find books with old labels. Make photocopies of these old designs; write the contents on them, or color them with markers. Cut them out and attach to your containers using craft glue. For an antiqued look, dip your labels in strong coffee or tea and let air-dry. Office supply stores are also a wonderful source for labels and tags. Another way to make beautiful tags is from aluminum foil cookie sheets—they look like sterling silver! Cut up the foil into interesting shapes such as leaves, stars, or diamonds. Use a dull pencil to write on the foil, and punch a hole in one corner with an office hole punch.

To finish the look, I like to tie something around the neck of the bottle or jar. There are many different materials you can use. My local craft store devotes an entire aisle to ribbons. My personal favorite is natural raffia, a grass from Madagascar that can be twisted, braided, dyed different colors, and tied in bows. I wrap it around the neck of jars and bottles several times and then tie it in a simple square knot. You can also tie something on the container that complements the contents: a cinnamon stick, a small bunch of herbs, or a wooden spoon for scooping out the contents. Make "necklaces" for your bottles using pretty beads, seeds, and spices. Using a sharp needle, string different items onto thread or dental floss and hang these around the neck of the container.

Fabric scraps can also be used to decorate your finished products. Tie a small square or circle around the neck of bottles or jar tops. Sew small sacks for your smaller products, such as lip gloss and fragrance. Drawstring muslin bags can become relaxing bath sacks: Fill with herbs or oatmeal, and hang them under the running water faucet of the tub.

You are the cosmetic manufacturer, and the packaging of your products should reflect this. Put your signature on every bottle, jar, and tin, and have fun sharing your creations!

DRYING HERBS AND FLOWERS

You can preserve fresh ingredients when they're in season to use throughout the year in your favorite beauty recipes. Dried ingredients have a more intense flavor and scent than fresh ingredients. In some recipes, such as those for scented oils, they're also preferred when you do not want any additional moisture introduced (moisture can cause bacteria to grow and spoil the end product).

The process of drying plants and peels for cosmetic use is similar to that for culinary use. (It differs from craft and floral use because the appearance of the flowers and herbs is not as important as the quality of the dried plant materials.) It is important for the plants to have been grown without any harmful chemicals, such as insecticides, which can remain on the leaves and flowers. Wash citrus fruits completely to remove any chemical preservatives from their skin. It is also important while drying substances to keep them from becoming dusty. You can prevent this by covering them with cheesecloth or placing them inside paper sacks with slits cut to allow air to circulate. You want to avoid any dirt and even small insects ending up in your cosmetic products. Once something is dry, it should be removed promptly and put in a clean container. If the herbs and flowers are hung for too long, you run the risk of their being contaminated and losing their usefulness as anything other than a decorative element.

The three main methods of drying are:

1. Air-drying
2. Oven-drying
3. Using a special appliance (microwave or food dehydrator).

The early morning is the best time to harvest your garden herbs and flowers—after the dew has dried but before the sun comes out and warms them. (The essential oils lose their quality when exposed to heat.) Plants grow from the inside out; the oldest leaves and flowers will be on the outside of the plant. Using sharp scissors, harvest your plants. Be careful to leave at least one-third of the plant so that it will continue to grow and produce. Flower petals should be picked after the flower has bloomed but before they drop to the ground. If you purchase fresh herbs and flowers, make sure they have been grown without the use of harmful insecticides, which remain on the plant. Wash your harvested items with cool water and pat dry with a clean towel. Group them by plant type and use the following drying methods to enjoy your harvest throughout the year!

Air-drying is the most popular and easiest method. Herbs and flowers are bunched together and simply hung upside down. Dark, dry, well-ventilated places work best. If the humidity is especially high where you live, you may want to use a small fan or heater in the room. Make small bunches—no more than one inch in diameter—for drying; if the bunches are too large, mildew may develop inside them. I use rubber bands to bind my bunches together because they contract as the plants dry. Hang these bunches upside down so that all the plant's "energy" flows to the head of the flower or herb; it also keeps the stems nice and straight. I screwed small cup hooks into the rafters of my garage and hang my plants from them. Wooden clothes-drying racks also work well, and they can be folded up when not in use. Clothes hangers are also good for hanging bunches on, especially if you're using an empty closet for drying. If you're drying many different types of herbs, you may want to tie small paper labels to the bunches. To prevent dust from contaminating your bunches, tie a large paper sack over them. Make sure to cut several slits in the bag to increase air circulation, and check the contents often to make sure they are drying.

When your herbs and flowers are crisp and dry, remove the buds and leaves from their stems and place in clean, dry containers. (Glass jars with screw-top lids work best.) For petals and peels you may want to use a drying screen or basket. I have a large, flat, round basket that I use for rose petals. Every time I walk by the basket I give the petals a little stir. In a couple of days they are perfectly dry. You can also make a drying screen from an old picture frame and clean window screening. Using a staple gun, secure a piece of screen to the underside of the frame. Baskets and screens are good for air-drying because they allow the air to circulate through the plant materials.

Using a conventional oven for drying plant materials is also a good method. It is quicker than air-drying, and the problem of dust is greatly reduced. Spread your flowers and herbs on a clean cookie sheet and place the sheet in the center of your oven. Use the lowest possible temperature setting—about 150 degrees Fahrenheit, or "Warm." Check every two to three hours. When your herbs or flowers are dry and crisp, let them cool completely and then store them in clean airtight jars.

Microwave ovens can also be used for drying herbs and flowers. Some manufacturers even list procedures for doing this in the owner's manual. This method works best for small batches of herbs, petals, and peels. What can take two weeks to air-dry can be done in as little as two minutes in the microwave! Every make and model of microwave varies slightly in how it dries, but here is the procedure I use: Place a cup of water in the far corner of the microwave. Lay a paper towel in the bottom of a microwave-safe baking dish. Lay a single layer of herbs or flower petals on the paper towel, cover with another paper towel, and place the dish in the microwave. Heat the plants for one minute on the lowest setting ("defrost" on my oven). Check and continue heating at thirty-second intervals. Stop if black spots form—that means you're burning them. When dry and crisp, let cool completely and then package in an airtight container.

Another special appliance that works well for drying herbs, flowers, and peels is a food dehydrator. Many of these come with instructions for drying plant materials, so check your owner's manual before starting. Using a food dehydrator works extremely well. It is quick and clean, and because it uses warm air to dry, the plants retain more of their scent and essential oils. It is air-drying without the worry of dust. I place whatever I want to dry on the drying racks and use a heat setting of 100 to 130 degrees Fahrenheit. I start my machine in the morning, and it is usually ready by the end of the day. But don't forget to turn off your dehydrator before leaving the house.

When storing your dried items, remember they are sensitive to heat and strong light. A cool, dark, dry cupboard is the best place for them. Canning jars and spice bottles with screw lids work best and can be reused. Always label your jars and date them. Freezing works well to store fresh herbs. Simply lay out the leaves on a piece of wax paper, roll up, and slip the roll into a resealable plastic bag to be put in the freezer. When using these frozen herbs, remove only what you need for the recipe and keep the rest frozen.

Dried herbs and flowers can be used in any recipe in place of fresh. The measuring rule of thumb is one-third the amount of dry to fresh; in other words, if your recipe calls for one cup of fresh lavender flowers, use one-third cup of dried flowers. Drying flowers, seeds, peels, and leaves when in season will give you a supply of ingredients to use in recipes all year long.

CREATING BEAUTIFUL GIFT BASKETS

There are a few simple tricks to creating the gorgeous and inviting baskets you see in so many catalogs and beauty boutiques. The most important step in creating a unique and personal gift is to choose a theme. I keep an idea file on hand for inspiration. It is filled with clippings from magazines and catalogs of finished baskets, color combinations, witty sayings and poems, nature photos, and gift ideas. I flip through this file before starting on a basket to get my creative juices flowing.

The theme can be very simple, such as the type of person the gift is for: your girlfriend, husband, daughter, or teacher. Or it can express a particular mood you are in: relaxing, uplifting, or romantic. Special events, such as graduation and holidays, also make wonderful basket themes.

Choose your basket to complement your gift theme. I use the term "basket" very loosely here. Any container can be used; in fact, I encourage you to use a wide variety. Import stores are a good place for unusual containers from around the world. I like to pick up baskets at tag sales and flea markets; after a good cleaning or coat of spray paint, they are ready to be filled. Other containers to try are terra-cotta pots and planters, aluminum and plastic buckets, large seashells, tote bags, brown paper sacks, wooden boxes, cosmetic bags, and ceramic bowls.

You will also need filling material—something to put in the bottom of the container so that the contents seem to fill the basket and so that the items do not touch one another. Filling material can be anything soft and pliable: tissue paper, shredded paper, popped popcorn, cotton batting, straw, raffia, dried flowers, or natural wood fibers.

Place a small amount of the filling material in the bottom of your container and place your gift items on top of it. Play with the arrangement until it pleases you. I like to tie small items such as bottles of essential oil or small brushes around the container or on the basket handle. You want the container to look as if it is very full, almost overflowing with gifts. The size of your container is very important. (A bit too small is better than too large because you want all the gifts to be visible.)

It isn't necessary, but many people like to "wrap" their gift basket in clear or printed cellophane wrap. I do this only if I am shipping the basket or having it delivered. In place of cellophane you can wrap several strands of raffia, jute, or fabric ribbon around the container to keep everything in place.

The final touch is to attach a large and festive bow or ornament to your package. Bows can be made from paper or fabric ribbon and decorated with dried flowers, nuts, spices, and herbs. A sprig of fresh flowers is a lovely addition, especially in the spring and summer months. If it is going to be a while before you give the basket, you may want to use water vials (available at craft and floral stores) to keep the flowers fresh.

Part of the fun in creating your own baskets is in making them uniquely yours. Throughout the book I will be giving you basket themes and ideas to go along with the recipes and products you are creating. I hope these ideas help to spark your imagination!

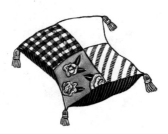

Winter Skin and Hair Care

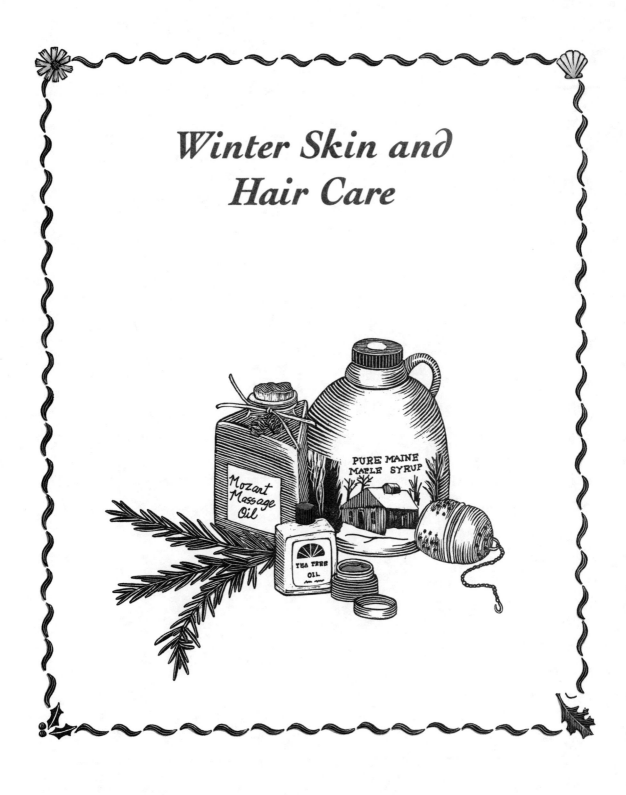

Winter is a wonderful time of year—holidays, warm fires, crisp brisk air, and, for many people, freshly fallen snow. Our choice of fresh produce is limited this time of year, but there are several excellent beauty ingredients ready to be discovered on your pantry shelves. Spices, natural oils, dried beans, and maple syrup are just a few of my favorite winter ingredients.

This season is also marked by colder, drier weather. We raise the heat indoors, which also dries the air. The colder temperature and lower humidity affect the condition of both your skin and hair. Even where the temperatures are milder, the humidity still drops in the winter months.

Winter is the one season when everyone needs a *good moisturizer!* Even if you have oily skin, you may need to start using one; if you have dry skin, you may want to use an extra-strength cream or lotion. The recipe for Winter Moisturizer on page 48 is a good one to try. Winter dryness strikes where your skin's oil glands are weakest. Cheeks, arms, and legs have almost no sebaceous oil glands and are therefore drier in winter months. The skin on your hands is thinner than in other places and needs extra protection and care. After washing your hands, always dry them thoroughly and use a good hand cream. Wearing gloves outdoors will also protect them and keep your skin soft.

We also wear more layers of clothes in the winter months. Elbows, knees, and feet are completely covered and usually forgotten until the spring. Clothing, shoes, and boots can cause friction that creates a buildup of thick skin. A good scrubbing with a natural loofah sponge or my Pine Nut Scrub on page 44 will help remove any problem skin that has developed.

Sun protection is also very important in winter, just as it is year-round. Many people forget to use sunscreen when outdoors, but sun reflects off snow and ice, so you can actually get double the sun exposure.

Protect your lips and wear a hat to protect your hair. Dry, chapped lips are often a result of bitter winter weather. Use a good protective lip balm when outdoors. Try to avoid licking your lips, which actually dries out your lips more, causing them to chap and crack. To gently exfoliate dry lips, cover them with a layer of light oil and using a warm, wet washcloth gently brush your lips. Brisk winds and low humidity are also hard on winter hair. Using a rich, deep hair conditioner is important to restore moisture to your hair. Try the Hot Oil Treatment for Winter Hair on page 69.

Practicing the art of massage is a perfect activity for a cold winter day spent indoors. Massage is relaxing, fun, and, depending on your choice of massage oil, it can also be very warming—especially in front of a fire. Try the Amorous Massage Oil on page 65, scented with vanilla and cinnamon. You'll also find it makes a perfect Valentine's Day gift!

Natural beauty products also make wonderful gifts for the holidays. Make up a special Merry Christmas Basket like the one on page 86, using your favorite yuletide scents such as pine and peppermint. Bath products are also great small presents to give when celebrating Hanukkah. See the basket on page 87. I also like to make up a few extra batches of colored bath salts to have on hand for last-minute hostess gifts, which are always appreciated.

For a description of common winter ingredients and where to find them, see page 16.

Black-Eyed Pea Cleanser

In the South, black-eyed peas are thought to bring luck in the New Year. They are high in protein, iron, and B vitamins. Finely ground, they make a gentle cleanser that is perfect for all skin types. Try other dried beans in this recipe such as pink azuki beans, red kidney beans, or black beans. Dried peas and beans are easy to find at any grocery store.

½ cup dried black-eyed peas

Preheat your oven to 400°F. Spread the beans out on a cookie sheet or baking pan and bake for 5 minutes to remove any moisture. Do not overbake. Let the beans cool completely.

Place the beans in a clean coffee or spice grinder and grind to a fine powder. Sift the ground beans using a flour sifter and discard any pieces that remain in the sifter. To use: Mix the bean powder with a little warm water in the palm of your hand to create a smooth cleansing cream. Massage the cream over your face, rinse with warm water, and pat dry.

Store any leftover cleanser in a clean, dry container.

Yield: 4 ounces

Lady Godiva Body Scrub

Lady Godiva was the wife of Earl Leofric of Mercia. As legend has it, she asked her husband to reduce the taxes for the people of Coventry. He agreed, but only if she would ride naked through the town. She asked the townspeople to remain indoors, and she rode covered only by her long hair. To prepare for her famous ride, I suspect she gave herself an all-over body scrub like this one so that her fleeting figure had a noble glow.

¼ cup granulated sugar
2 tablespoons light vegetable oil
2 tablespoons fresh whole milk

Mix together all the ingredients into a smooth cream.

To use: Before bathing, gently massage the mixture all over your body to increase circulation and remove dry, flaky skin. Rinse your skin with warm water and moisturize well.

Save any extra in the refrigerator but discard it if the milk sours.

Yield: 4 ounces, enough for 1 whole body treatment

Pine Nut Scrub

½ cup pine nuts
2 tablespoons light oil (for dry skin) or 2 tablespoons spring water (for oily skin)

Pine nuts, which are high-fat, grow on pine or pignon trees and are found inside the pine cone. These smooth, soft, white nuts make an excellent skin-softening scrub that can be used all over your body and is gentle enough for sensitive skin.

In a blender or food processor, place the pine nuts and oil or water, and process until finely ground. Use the grainy mixture to cleanse your skin. Store any leftover scrub in the refrigerator.

Yield: 4 ounces, enough for 1 whole body treatment

Cognac Astringent

Cognac is a type of grape brandy distilled in a town in France with the same name, located between Saintes and Angoulême near the Bay of Biscay. It makes an excellent astringent for everyday use. If you prefer an unscented product, simply substitute more distilled water for the orange flower water.

3 tablespoons distilled water
3 tablespoons orange flower water
1 tablespoon Cognac

Mix together all the ingredients. Place in a container with a lid so the alcohol will not evaporate. To use: Apply to your skin with a clean cotton ball. Store in a cool, dark, dry place.

Yield: 3½ ounces

Pine Toner

Fresh pine needles are easy to find this time of year. This fragrant toner is perfect for all skin types. Pine water is slightly astringent and will improve your circulation, giving your complexion a healthy winter glow! The subtle scent of pine also produces a feeling of tranquility. For gift-giving I like to place a sprig of fresh pine inside the bottle and nestle the toner in a basket filled with fresh pine needles and pine cone scales.

1 cup fresh pine needles
1 cup distilled water
¼ cup witch hazel

Place the pine needles in a small saucepan on the stove and cover with the water. Bring the water to a boil, then remove the pan from the heat.

Allow the pine water to cool completely. Strain off the pine needles and discard. Add the witch hazel and stir well. Pour the toner into a clean bottle.

Apply to your skin with a clean cotton ball. Do not rinse. Store in a cool, dark, dry place.

Yield: 8 ounces

Florida Grapefruit Freshener

Peel from 1 medium-size grapefruit
  (approximately ½ cup)
1 vitamin C tablet
1 cup boiling water

Florida is famous for its citrus orchards. Each Christmas I receive a box of gorgeous fresh grapefruits from a good friend in this southern state. When I make this recipe, the scent from the grapefruit peel is an instant energizer! You can substitute lemon and orange peels for the grapefruit peel, or try a combination of all three.

Place the grapefruit peel in a small ceramic or glass bowl. Dissolve the vitamin C tablet in the boiling water and pour the solution over the peels. Allow the mixture to cool completely. When cool, strain the liquid into a clean container.

To use: Apply to the skin with a clean cotton ball or spray bottle. Store in a cool, dark, dry place.

Yield: 8 ounces

Carpe Diem Splash

½ cup rosewater
1 cup white wine
2 bay leaves
6 clove buds
3 black peppercorns

Carpe diem is Latin for "Seize the day!" Use this spicy after-bath splash to make your mornings more invigorating. It is mildly astringent and acidic, and will help restore your skin's natural acid mantle. Make sure to moisturize well after using the splash because it can be drying.

Place all the ingredients in a small saucepan or microwave-safe container. Bring the mixture to a boil. Remove from the heat and allow to cool. Pour the mixture into a clean container and let it sit for at least 2 weeks (the longer the better). Strain the bath splash and rebottle it in a clean container with a tight-fitting lid.

To use: Spray or splash on the body after bathing. Store in a cool, dark, dry place.

Yield: 10 ounces

WORKOUT BASKET

New Year's is a time of resolutions, and one of the most popular is to exercise regularly. (I know. I make it myself each year.) Give that special friend or loved one a sign of support by creating a simple workout basket as a gift. Put together a few items that can be used as a reward after an especially tough day or can be kept in the gym locker.

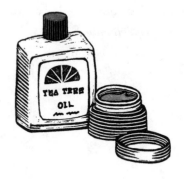

Suggested items to include:

Scented shower gels
(see April Showers gels on page 116)

Marathon Massage Oil (page 233)

New gym towel

Carpe Diem Splash (page 46)

Foot Powder (page 187)

Exercise video or cassette tape

Use a nylon duffle bag or plastic tote basket for your container and fill with active, healthy items. Make sure you use plastic nonbreakable containers for the shower items. You may also want to include some small snacks (nuts, granola bars, juice boxes). Clip pictures and quotes from magazines and paste the collection, along with a few motivational statements, onto a piece of heavy construction paper. Your "collage" can be hung on the wall or inside a locker for inspiration.

Sleeping Beauty Cream

1 tablespoon grated beeswax
1 teaspoon vitamin E oil
¼ cup light sesame oil
¼ cup orange flower water
Pinch of borax powder

One of my daughter's favorite fairy tales is Charles Perrault's story of a beautiful princess cast into a deep sleep by a jealous fairy's curse. She can only be awakened by a kiss of true love. This cream recipe contains orange flower water. It gives the cream a relaxing scent that will help you sleep. When you awake, your skin will be full of moisture and glowing with beauty.

Mix together the beeswax, vitamin E oil, and sesame oil. Heat gently until the beeswax is melted. Combine the orange flower water and borax powder, and heat until very warm. Pour the warm water into the oil mixture and stir well. Continue to stir, or pour the whole mixture into an electric blender and blend for 1 minute. Pour the cream into a clean container and allow the mixture to cool completely. Store in a cool, dry place.

Yield: 4 ounces

Winter Moisturizer

2 tablespoons apricot kernel oil
¼ cup walnut oil
¼ cup stearic acid powder
½ teaspoon fresh baking soda
1 tablespoon aloe vera gel
1 cup water

We all need a good moisturizer in winter, and you may want to give this one a try. It is light, fluffy, and easily absorbed, and it doesn't leave an oily film on the skin. It contains stearic acid powder, which gives the cream a lighter feel and texture than beeswax. Stearic acid is a natural butter acid obtained from fats and oils. I purchase it from chemical supply companies. Craft stores also carry it because it is used in candle making to create a longer-burning candle.

Combine the oils and stearic acid powder in a heat-resistant container.

Combine the baking soda, aloe vera gel, and water in another heat-resistant container.

Heat the oil mixture in a water bath until the mixture is a clear liquid and all the stearic acid powder is melted.

Heat the water solution until just boiling (in the same water bath or 1–2 minutes in the microwave). Slowly add ⅓ of the water solution to the oil mixture and stir. The combination will foam slightly as carbon dioxide is released.

Pour this mixture into a blender and stir. Add the rest of the water mixture in a slow, steady stream and blend on high. The mixture will be a white fluffy cream. Spoon the cream into a clean container and allow to cool completely.

Massage a small amount of the cream on your face and neck. Store the cream in a cool, dry place.

Yield: 12 ounces

Eggnog Lotion

A light lubricating lotion, this egg-based moisturizer is a skin saver during the holiday season and can be used for both face and body application. Egg yolks make a great natural treatment because they are rich in natural lecithin, which is often called "nature's emulsifier." An emulsifier holds together two unmixable liquids, such as oil and water, and has a smooth, creamy texture. You can also pour one or two tablespoons of this lotion into your bath for a rich, relaxing soak.

2 egg yolks
½ cup heavy cream or half-and-half
1 tablespoon rum
¼ cup light oil (canola, almond, and walnut work well)

In a blender, mix together the egg yolks, cream, and rum until well blended. With the blender running, slowly add the oil in a thin stream until well combined. Pour the creamy lotion into a clean container and store in the refrigerator.

Yield: 8 ounces

Great Expectations Cream

¼ cup cocoa butter
1 teaspoon light sesame oil
1 teaspoon apricot kernel oil
1 teaspoon vitamin E oil

When I was pregnant, I used this rich cream on my stomach, chest, and legs to keep my skin soft and supple. I like to think it helps reduce your chances of getting stretch marks (but heredity plays a key role in your skin's fate). Pampering yourself is always a good idea, and massaging this cream into your skin feels wonderful! It also relieves the itchiness that many women experience from their skin stretching during pregnancy. I used the cream after showering while my skin was still warm and damp. It also makes a nice baby shower gift for a special friend.

Place all the ingredients in an ovenproof glass container and gently heat until the cocoa butter is melted and the oils are well mixed. Pour into a clean container and allow the cream to cool completely. Store in a cool, dry place.

Yield: 2½ ounces

Cocoa Body Lotion

This is a light lotion, perfect for massaging into warm skin after a bath or shower. Between uses the cocoa butter may harden. Simply place the container in a cup of warm water before using to gently remelt the cocoa butter and warm the oil, then shake to reblend.

2 tablespoons grated cocoa butter
2 tablespoons castor oil
2 tablespoons vodka

Mix together the cocoa butter and castor oil, and heat gently to melt the cocoa butter. This can be done in the microwave or in a water bath. Add the vodka and stir well. Allow the mixture to cool completely and stir once more to blend the lotion.

Yield: 3 ounces

Venus Facial Steam

Venus was the Roman goddess of love and beauty (the Greeks named her Aphrodite). In what may have been the world's first beauty contest, Paris (a prince of Troy) selected her—over Hera and Athena—as the most beautiful goddess. This is a simple, yet effective facial steam that can also be used as a mild astringent when cool. Weekly use will result in beautiful healthy skin worthy of any goddess.

½ cup dry white wine
½ cup witch hazel

Pour the wine and witch hazel into a small saucepan or microwave-safe bowl and bring to a boil. You may add a drop or two of your favorite essential oil or dried herbs. Note: If you have especially dry skin, add ½ cup water to dilute the mixture. Place the mixture in a shallow dish and gently steam your face. (Follow directions for facial steaming on page 195.)

Yield: 8 ounces, enough for 1 facial steam

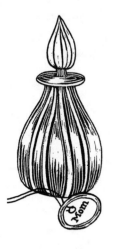

NEW MOTHER BASKET

Becoming a new mother is one of the most exciting and wonderful times in a woman's life. It is also a time that calls for pampering, as nothing can be as physically demanding as a new mother's schedule.

Suggested items to include:

Essential oil of lavender
Great Expectations Cream (page 50)
Dream Pillow (page 77)
Scented Dusting Powder (page 224)
New Year's Baby Bath (page 57)
Orange flower water

Line a pretty basket with a flannel baby blanket and fill with beauty items. Include a blank notebook or diary to record those precious first days and to keep track of feeding and sleeping schedules. Sprinkle some dried lavender in the bottom of the basket. The scent is very calming to both mother and baby. (In Australia, lavender oil is added to the bathwater to calm colicky babies.) The orange flower water can be added to a cup of warm milk (one teaspoon) for a fragrant and relaxing evening drink. Cut a long strip of gingham or floral fabric and tie up the basket with a large pretty bow.

Madzoon
Facial Mask

¼ cup plain yogurt

*T*he first commercial yogurt dairy in the United States was the Colombo Dairy in Metuen, Massachusetts. In 1929 it produced a product called Madzoon, the Armenian name for yogurt. Plain yogurt is one of my favorite beauty ingredients — I always have a tubful in my refrigerator. It is mildly acidic, which is perfect for removing surface impurities and restoring the skin's own protective acid mantle.

Spread the yogurt over your skin (it can be used all over the body) and let sit for 15–20 minutes. Rinse or shower with warm water and pat your skin dry. Remember to use a rich moisturizer or oil, such as almond or jojoba oil. So simple and so effective.

Yield: 2 ounces, enough for 1 facial mask

Cherimoya
Facial Mask

½ cherimoya fruit, peeled and seeds discarded

*C*herimoyas, an edible fruit, grow wild in Peru and are available to us during the winter months. They are often called the "custard fruit" because of their white creamy interior. The fresh pulp tastes like a mixture of pineapple and banana, and makes an excellent facial treatment because it's so moisturizing and soothing to dry winter skin.

Mash the fruit into a smooth paste. You may add a bit of powdered milk or cornstarch, if you wish, to firm up the mixture. Spread over clean skin and let sit for 10–15 minutes. Rinse with warm water and pat dry. Follow with a rich moisturizer or light oil.

Yield: Approximately 4 ounces, enough for 1 facial mask

Egyptian Facial Mask

1 egg, beaten
½ teaspoon olive oil
1 tablespoon flour
¼ teaspoon sea salt
1 tablespoon whole milk

In 3000 B.C., *Egyptian women troubled by blemishes treated their complexions with a mask of whipped ostrich eggs, olive oil, flour, sea salt, and milk. Sound exotic? While ostrich eggs may be hard to come by, the other ingredients are still basic home beauty staples that can be found in any grocery store. Try this simple ancient mask recipe for soft, smooth skin.*

Mix together all the ingredients until creamy and well blended. Spread the mixture over your face and neck, and leave on for 15 minutes. Rinse well with cool water and pat dry.

Yield: 2 ounces, enough for 1 facial mask

Mardi Gras Mask

1 tablespoon French green clay
   (see page 109)
1 tablespoon orange flower water
1 teaspoon pineapple juice
¼ ripe banana, mashed

Mardi Gras, which means "Fat Tuesday" in French, is the noisy, colorful celebration that ends a month-long carnival season. This winter celebration is the perfect inspiration for a light, amusing mask that is perfect for all skin types. Spread this fragrant mixture over clean skin, put on some lively music, and enjoy yourself!

Mix together all the ingredients in a small bowl with a fork until you have a smooth paste. Spread the mixture on clean skin (it can be used on both the face and body) and let sit for 15 minutes. Rinse with tepid water and pat dry.

Yield: 2 ounces, enough for 1 facial mask

Martha Washington Mask

During the French and Indian War (which began in 1754), George Washington met and fell in love with pretty Martha Custis at a dance. Washington married Martha, a rich widow with children, in 1759. From across the dance floor he must have noticed her famous complexion, which she maintained by using this simple facial treatment. Honey is a natural humectant, and vinegar helps restore your skin's own natural acid level, which is so important for healthy skin.

1 egg, separated
1 teaspoon honey
¼ teaspoon apple cider vinegar

Beat the egg white until frothy. Mix together the egg yolk, honey, and vinegar. Fold this into the egg white. Spread the entire mixture over your face and neck. Leave the mask on your skin for 15–20 minutes, then rinse with warm water and pat dry. Refrigerate any leftover mask but discard after a few days.

Yield: 2 ounces, enough for 1 facial mask

Maple Nut Lip Gloss

Here is a delightfully simple, light lip gloss. It's a good substitute for plain old petroleum jelly and has a slightly sweet flavor. I like to wear it all by itself, but it can also be used over your favorite lip color for greater shine.

1 teaspoon grated cocoa butter
¼ teaspoon grated beeswax
½ teaspoon coconut oil
½ teaspoon walnut oil
¼ teaspoon pure maple syrup
⅛ teaspoon vitamin E oil

Combine the cocoa butter, beeswax, and oils, and heat gently until melted. Remove from the heat source and stir in the maple syrup and vitamin E oil. Stir well until all the ingredients are combined and let cool completely. Spoon into a small clean container with a lid.

Yield: ½ ounce

Matterhorn Lip Balm

1 teaspoon vegetable shortening
½ teaspoon castor oil
½ teaspoon grated beeswax
½ teaspoon almond oil
⅛ teaspoon vitamin E oil

One of my all-time favorite vacations was a trip to Europe in 1987, during which my husband and I visited the charming town of Zermatt, Switzerland. I felt like Heidi of the mountains: The close-up view of the snow-capped Matterhorn took my breath away. The air was cold and crisp, and I was grateful to have this rich lip balm to protect me from the drying wind that blew in the mountains. Vitamin E helps protect your lips, keeping them healthy and full of moisture.

Mix together all the ingredients in a heat-resistant container. Gently heat the mixture until the shortening and beeswax are melted. Stir the mixture well and allow to cool completely. When cool, spoon into a clean container and enjoy.

Yield: ½ ounce

Chocolate Lip Gloss

1½ teaspoons grated cocoa butter
½ teaspoon coconut oil
⅛ teaspoon vitamin E oil
¼ teaspoon grated chocolate or
    3 small chocolate chips (I like
    to use milk chocolate ones)

From the colorful fruits of the cacao tree come the raw ingredients for chocolate. The two main substances obtained from the wrinkly pods are cocoa butter and unsweetened chocolate (sold as bitter or baking chocolate). This lip gloss, made from blending together cocoa butter and chocolate, is an excellent lip conditioner with a mildly sweet taste. It also makes a terrific Valentine's Day present. You can give your sweetheart lots of chocolate kisses without all the calories! I like to wrap this lip gloss in aluminum foil so that it resembles a large Hershey's candy kiss.

In a double boiler or the microwave oven, heat the cocoa butter, coconut oil, and vitamin E oil gently until melted. Stir in the chocolate and keep stirring until melted and well blended. Pour into a small lip gloss container and allow to cool completely before using.

Yield: ½ ounce

New Year's Baby Bath

¼ cup nonfat dry milk
¼ cup whole dry buttermilk
1 tablespoon cornstarch
1 drop orange oil (optional)

This gentle milk bath will leave your baby's tender skin soft and silky. Milk is rich in fat and lactic acid, and both help soften and hydrate skin. Prepare an extra portion of this treatment for yourself because people of all ages can benefit from this rich, relaxing natural bath. You may even want to package this bath powder by making your own bath envelopes to give as gifts. (See the pattern on page 243.) Use pretty wrapping paper and fill each envelope with ¼ cup of bath powder. Label the outside with the contents and a short, sweet note.

Mix together all the ingredients and pour into a clean container or resealable plastic bag.

To use: Pour ¼ cup of the bath powder into a full tub or 1 tablespoon into a small baby bathtub.

Yield: 4 ounces, enough for 2 baths

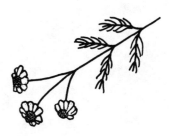

Sensuous Scented Bath Oils

½ cup light oil (olive, almond, macadamia, light sesame, apricot kernel, or your favorite)
Essential oils—see combinations below

Unique scented bath oils are super simple to create but make very impressive gifts! Select your favorite beauty oil—olive, sesame, almond, macadamia, or apricot kernel—and add a few drops of an essential oil combination listed below. Use the mixture before showering, in your bathwater, or as an after-bath moisturizer. Have fun experimenting with different scent combinations and their effects.

Pour the oil into a clean container and add the essential oils a drop at a time (many oils come packaged in drop dispensers). Shake gently to blend. Store in a cool, dark, dry place.

Some essential oil combinations:

KINDLE THE SPIRIT:
5 drops essential oil of lemon
5 drops essential oil of lavender
3 drops essential oil of peppermint

RELAX THE MIND:
5 drops essential oil of jasmine
5 drops essential oil of chamomile
5 drops essential oil of sandalwood

AWAKEN YOUR CREATIVITY:
5 drops essential oil of basil
5 drops essential oil of rosemary
3 drops essential oil of lavender
2 drops essential oil of frankincense

Yield: 4 ounces

Candy Cane Bath Salts

*B*oth of my daughters love candy canes. During the holidays they enjoy helping me create these scented bath salts. The red and white colors and peppermint scent always conjure up Christmas cheer for us. Peppermint can be very stimulating, so do not use these in the late evening before going to bed or you may have trouble falling asleep.

2 cups Epsom salts
½ cup rock salt or sea salt
4–5 drops peppermint oil
2–3 drops red food coloring

Place 1 cup of the Epsom salts and ¼ cup of rock salt in a mixing bowl or resealable plastic bag. Add 2–3 drops of peppermint oil and mix until evenly distributed.

Place the remaining 1 cup of Epsom salts and ¼ cup of rock salt in a separate bowl or bag. Add the food coloring and mix until the color is evenly distributed and you are pleased with the shade of red. Add 2–3 drops of peppermint oil and stir well.

In a large jar or clear bottle—I like to use spring water bottles—layer the white salts and red salts. You want to create a striped effect, like a candy cane. Place the top on your container and tie with a big bow and a few real candy canes.

Yield: 20 ounces

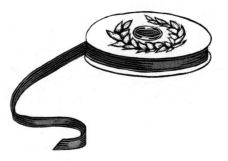

Sugar
and Spice
Bath Mix

½ cup baking soda
2 tablespoons sugar
1 teaspoon ground cinnamon
½ teaspoon ground ginger
¼ teaspoon ground cloves

Fill an old-fashioned sugar bowl or shaker with this spicy mixture and place it next to your tub. Cinnamon, cloves, and ginger are all antiseptic and stimulating spices. They will help boost your circulation. Sugar is often used as a substitute for glycerin in bath products. It will cleanse your skin and act as an antioxidant. If you have hard water, baking soda will soften it; it also acts as a mild skin cleanser.

Mix together all the ingredients until well blended. To use: Add 2 tablespoons of the bath mix to a warm tub of water. Store the mixture in a clean, dry container.

Yield: 5 ounces, enough for 2 to 3 baths

Greta Garbo
Bath

3 chamomile tea bags
3 fresh oranges

Greta Garbo was the Swedish beauty who became famous for her portrayal of mysterious women and led a reclusive life. Her now famous line, "I want to be alone," from the movie Grand Hotel *became a trademark, as did her luminous alabaster skin. During her baths Greta would often sip chamomile tea and eat fresh dates. She also loved oranges, which were a rare luxury in Stockholm where Garbo was raised. Oranges are full of vitamin C, which is essential for healthy, glowing skin. On your way to becoming a* femme fatale, *try soaking in this exquisite chamomile and orange bath that Garbo would have loved to spend her private moments in.*

Tie the tea bags under the pour spout on your bathtub and start filling the tub with warm water. Slice the fresh oranges and float them in the tub. Hang a DO NOT DISTURB sign on the bathroom door and slip into the aromatic waters. Relax and contemplate the fragrance of the citrus fruit and chamomile.

Yield: enough for 1 bath treatment

Color Therapy Baths

Using color in the bath is an exciting way to relax your body, balance your mind, and energize your spirit. Quite simply, color is visible light energy, and it can be used almost anywhere to create or enhance a particular mood. Try packaging several of these bath waters together to give as a set. I like to use small test tubes with stoppers (available at chemical and medical supply stores) to hold each color bath. You can also scent the waters to heighten their therapeutic effects. After bathing, extend the color mood by using colored towels and clothing or bedding.

Food coloring of your choice, not to exceed ½ teaspoon
1 tablespoon water
1 tablespoon glycerin
1 tablespoon liquid soap

Red: A red bath gives you courage, power, and strength. It can help you when you are feeling tired or when you have a big day ahead of you. It can also warm you up if you're chilled. In both the bath and the boardroom, red has become the new "power" color.

Orange: An orange bath can really heighten your mood and impart a feeling of independence. This is another great color to try in the morning when you need an extra boost. An orange bath sets a positive, productive tone for the rest of the day.

Yellow: A yellow bath can be soothing if you are feeling nervous or tense about a big meeting or test. Yellow helps sharpen and focus your mind while increasing your confidence. Yellow is the color of the sun and therefore a positive-energy color!

Green: A green bath represents the color of nature and will help restore in you a feeling of balance and harmony. A green bath is recommended in the evening for relaxation and peace of mind.

Blue: The color blue, like the ocean or sky, suggests serenity or calm. Blue is my favorite color to bathe in during the evening since it helps me sleep better, though I find that a blue bath quiets my mind and relaxes my nerves at any time.

Violet: A violet bath will energize your spirit and creative powers. Violet is considered the artist's primary color. Try a violet bath before tackling a big project or to gain a new perspective on an existing task.

Mix together all the ingredients and pour into a clean bottle. To use: Draw a warm bath, add the color bath to the water, and stir to distribute. Be careful when adding color to your bath; the undiluted color could stain.

Yield: 1½ ounces, enough for 1 bath

THE PERFECT MASSAGE

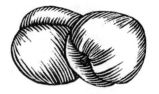

For an ideal massage environment, there are three factors to consider: the scene, the massage surface, and the massage oil. Careful selection in these three areas will give you (and your partner) the ultimate massage experience.

The scene or location you choose for the massage should be quiet and warm. The surrounding colors should be soft and natural; pastel shades are best. Use natural sunlight or candlelight (no bright or fluorescent lights, please). Relaxing instrumental music can be played in the background at a low volume.

The massage surface should be comfortable but firm. Professional massage tables work best, but even the floor is a good surface and can be made more comfortable with a thick blanket, an exercise mat, or a comforter. Unless you have a very firm mattress or futon, don't use a bed. Most beds are too soft for an effective massage because they absorb the pressure intended for the body.

An oil or lotion will undoubtedly enhance the massage experience. Scented oils can be used to create or change a mood, so ask your partner beforehand what scents he or she prefers. Use a very small amount of oil; you should be able to massage the whole body using about one tablespoon.

(continued)

Here are a few more guidelines to follow:

- Once you begin the massage, keep your hand in contact with your partner's body. Use natural breaks in the flow of the massage to rest or get more oil. A break might occur, for example, when you have finished the back and are moving on to the legs or arms.

- Add interest to the massage by varying the pressure you use from light to strong. Your partner should tell you if you are applying too much pressure.

- Use slow movements to relax and calm your partner, and brisk movements to stimulate or invigorate.

- To give an effective massage you need to be calm, relaxed, and unhurried. A full body massage, properly given, can take up to one hour.

- After the massage, allow your partner to rest and slowly get up when he or she desires.

Mozart Massage Oil

The great musical genius of Wolfgang Amadeus Mozart, an eighteenth-century Austrian composer, lives on to this day. I've found that Mozart's work creates the perfect musical background for this stimulating massage oil. The oil contains frankincense, a resin extracted from small leafy trees found in the Middle East and North Africa. Frankincense is believed to contain a psychoactive chemical that stimulates the subconscious. Perhaps this massage oil will help to bring out your partner's genius, too.

¼ cup almond oil
5 black peppercorns
1 teaspoon dried rosemary
2–3 drops essential oil of frankincense

Place the almond oil, peppercorns, and rosemary in a heat-resistant container and warm gently—do not boil. Let the mixture cool completely, strain, and add the frankincense oil. Pour into a clean bottle with a stopper. Try placing a sprig of dried rosemary inside the bottle.

Yield: 2 ounces

Amorous Massage Oil

This is my favorite massage oil recipe and one that I introduced to readers in my first book, Natural Beauty at Home. *I have received so many letters from happy couples who have used it that I've decided to include it again. The subtle spicy scent seems to appeal to everyone, and the scent of cinnamon is believed to be an aphrodisiac. (From all accounts, it is!) Pour this into a pretty red bottle and add a gold ribbon for a special valentine. The gift of a good massage is always welcome.*

½ cup light oil (canola, almond, safflower)
½ teaspoon ground cinnamon
½ teaspoon vanilla extract

Mix together all the ingredients. Let the mixture sit for several hours to allow the oil to absorb the cinnamon and vanilla. To remove any solids in the oil, pour the mixture into a clean jar or bottle through a funnel lined with a coffee filter. Cover your container and enjoy. For a stronger scent, place a cinnamon stick and/or a piece of vanilla bean inside the container.

Yield: 4 ounces

Virtual Reality Massage Oil

1 teaspoon dried basil
1 teaspoon dried rosemary
1 tablespoon grated or sliced
   grapefruit peel
½ cup walnut oil

The scents of basil and rosemary stimulate the mind and help crystallize your thoughts. This massage oil is perfect for deep thinkers, visionaries, and people who use a computer all day. Whether you are surfing the Internet or developing a new project, this energizing oil will enhance your productivity. Rub a small amount of it between your hands until warm, then place your palms over your eyelids. As you relax and focus on the scent and warmth of the oil, you should gradually feel refreshed and revived, ready to take on any intellectual challenge!

Combine all the ingredients in a heat-resistant container and warm gently—do not boil. Let the mixture cool completely, then pour into a clean jar and let sit for at least 1 week. Strain and bottle. A few pieces of dried grapefruit peel tied in knots (before drying) or dried rosemary look pretty floating in the bottle.

Yield: 4 ounces

Wasabi Massage Oil

½ cup light vegetable oil
¼ teaspoon wasabi powder or paste

*M*y friend Allie first introduced me to wasabi, a spicy Asian condiment. I am now a big fan and use it as a key ingredient in this wonderful massage oil. Wasabi, or Japanese horseradish, grows only in Japan, and it's extremely pungent and spicy. Fresh wasabi is hard to find outside of Japan, but powdered and paste forms are easily attainable. Added to a light oil, it creates a stimulating and warming massage oil that is perfect on a cold winter day.

Mix together the vegetable oil and wasabi and stir well to blend. Pour the oil into a clean container with a tight-fitting lid.

Yield: 4 ounces

Lullaby Oil

1 chamomile tea bag (make sure they're 100 percent chamomile flowers)
½ cup sweet almond oil
5 drops essential oil of lavender

*T*he scent of lavender and chamomile has been proven as effective for inducing drowsiness as sleep medications, and without any of the harmful side effects. This massage oil is the perfect antidote to even the worst case of insomnia. You can add a tablespoon to an evening bath or use it after bathing to moisturize your skin. Sweet dreams!

Place the chamomile tea bag in a small saucepan or microwave-safe container. Pour the almond oil over the tea bag and gently warm the oil for a few minutes—do not boil. Allow the oil to cool, then remove the tea bag and add the lavender oil. Pour the mixture into a clean bottle with a tight-fitting lid. A stem or two of dried lavender looks pretty floating inside the bottle.

Yield: 4 ounces

MASSAGE-AT-HOME BASKET

A good massage in itself is a wonderful gift since your time and energy are focused on pleasing and relaxing someone else. A massage basket is a nice accompaniment to a promised massage for your partner, or a way of providing the essentials for another busy couple. I like to give this basket as a wedding present — with a couple of beautiful champagne flutes and a good bottle of bubbly tucked inside, of course!

Suggested items to include:

Mozart Massage Oil (page 65)
Scented candle or fireplace potpourri
Amorous Massage Oil (page 65)
Classical music or Relaxation Tape
(page 168)

Line a round basket with some natural muslin or cheesecloth and stitch in place with linen thread. Fill the basket with cotton wool or batting and wrap each present in cotton fabric. I like to use cheesecloth from the grocery store; it can be reused, and its sheer texture softly wraps each item. Make a beautiful gift card and hand-print a meaningful poem or quote inside.

Hot Oil Treatment for Winter Hair

Deep conditioning is important for dry and brittle winter hair. Once a week treat your tresses to a hot oil treatment to keep them looking their best. Olive oil increases your hair's strength and flexibility. This is especially important if you use heated styling tools such as blow dryers, curling irons, or electric rollers that can cause damage to your hair.

Place the olive oil in a blender and carefully add the boiling water. Blend on high speed until the oil has broken up into tiny droplets. Work into your dry hair, massaging well all over. Put a shower cap or plastic bag over your hair and wrap your head in a towel. Leave on for 20 minutes, then shampoo and condition as usual.

Yield: 4 ounces, enough for 1 treatment

¼ cup olive oil
¼ cup boiling distilled water

Quebec Maple Syrup Hair Conditioner

Maple syrup is made from the sweet sap of certain species of maple trees, the sugar maple being the chief source. Vermont and New York are the main producers of maple syrup in the United States, but the Canadian province of Quebec produces more than both these states.

Maple sap is a colorless watery solution that contains sugar, various acids, and salts. It takes thirty-five to forty-five gallons of sap to make just one gallon of syrup. The amber color we are accustomed to seeing develops as the sap is processed. Pure maple syrup is a treat for dry, damaged hair. It is a natural humectant, similar to honey and molasses. It does wonders for dry hair, restoring lost moisture and giving it extra body and shine.

Pour the syrup onto clean, dry hair and massage into the scalp and ends. Wrap your hair in plastic wrap or

½ cup pure maple syrup

use a plastic shower cap. Cover the plastic with a towel and leave the syrup on your hair for 20–30 minutes. Rinse well with warm water.

Yield: 4 ounces, enough for 1 treatment

Winter Hair Conditioner

1 tablespoon vegetable shortening
1 tablespoon castor oil
½ cup water
1 teaspoon white vinegar
1 teaspoon glycerin

Cold, dry winter weather can be hard on the hair. Coming and going from warm houses and offices to the frigid weather conditions outside can cause moisture to be drawn from the scalp, leaving your hair dry and brittle. This oil-rich conditioner can help restore lost moisture and protect your hair from the cold air. It leaves hair soft and easy to comb. (Glycerin, by the way, can be found in most pharmacies.)

Mix together the shortening and castor oil and warm gently until the shortening is liquefied. In a separate container, mix together the water, vinegar, and glycerin. Warm this mixture but do not boil. By hand or using a blender slowly beat the oil mixture into the water mixture. Allow the conditioner to cool completely. To use: Apply 1 tablespoon to just-shampooed hair, rinse well, and dry and style as usual.

Yield: 6 ounces

Shampoo Enhancers

*M*ake a batch of Basic Shampoo (recipe below) or alter an inexpensive mild shampoo with these shampoo "enhancers." It's very easy to create shampoo with simple, natural ingredients that will give your hair added body, bounce, and luster.

BASIC SHAMPOO

This is my recipe for Basic Shampoo from Natural Beauty at Home.
½ cup water
½ cup liquid soap
½ teaspoon light vegetable oil (omit if you have very oily hair)

Mix together all the ingredients. Pour the shampoo into a clean squeeze bottle or plastic container. Shampoo as you would normally and rinse well with cool water.

Yield: 8 ounces

ENHANCERS

For Normal Hair

Beer: Place 1 cup of beer in a saucepan and boil until reduced to ¼ cup. Add this to 1 cup of Basic Shampoo and stir well.

Egg: Mix together 1 tablespoon of Basic Shampoo and 1 raw egg. Use this mixture to shampoo your hair.

For Oily Hair

Lemon juice: Add 2 tablespoons of fresh lemon juice to 1 cup of Basic Shampoo and stir well.

Aloe vera gel: Add ¼ cup of aloe vera gel to 1 cup of Basic Shampoo and stir well.

For Dry Hair

Honey: Mix together 1 tablespoon of honey and 1 tablespoon of Basic Shampoo.

Jojoba oil: Add 2 tablespoons of jojoba oil and ¼ cup water to 1 cup of Basic Shampoo. Shampoo as usual and rinse well with warm water. If hair seems too oily, shampoo once more with 1 teaspoon of plain shampoo.

Dandruff Treatments

Dry indoor climates and cold outside temperatures can create dry, flaky scalps—known as dandruff. It is the most common scalp problem and easily cured. Serious cases of scalp dryness, however, should be treated by a physician.

For an Oily, Flaky Scalp

*2 tablespoons apple cider vinegar
  or fresh lemon juice
2 tablespoons distilled water
2 tablespoons olive oil*

Mix together all the ingredients and massage into your scalp. Leave on for 20 minutes before shampooing.

Yield: 3 ounces, enough for 1 treatment

For a Dry, Flaky Scalp

2 tablespoons jojoba oil
¼ teaspoon tea tree oil

Combine the 2 oils and massage into clean wet hair. Leave on for 10 minutes, then shampoo out.

Yield: 1 ounce, enough for 1 treatment

Chateau Nail Polish

1 tablespoon pure olive oil
½ tablespoon talc or powdered white clay

My friend Leslie brought back this recipe for me from a recent trip to France, during which she visited the Château d'Estublon in Font Vieille. At the château they produce a variety of fine wines and olive oils. Her host, M. Eric Lombrage, shared this French beauty tip for healthy nails using fresh olive oil. By massaging this mixture into clean nails, you will improve your hand's circulation while promoting new nail growth. The talc or clay enhances the nail's natural luster and works as a gentle polish.

Mix together the olive oil and talc into a smooth cream. If the mixture seems too thick, add a bit more olive oil.

To use: Massage a small amount into your nails and cuticles. Wipe off any excess with a soft cloth or cotton pad and buff lightly for a soft natural glow. Save any extra in a small container with a lid or cover with plastic wrap.

Yield: ½ ounce

Molasses Nail Soak

1/4 cup warm water
2 tablespoons molasses

Pure molasses made from the juice of fresh sugarcane can be used as a soak to soften cuticles and strengthen and condition nails before a manicure. Like honey, molasses is an excellent natural humectant that helps restore lost moisture to the skin and nails. (Don't worry—it won't leave your hands all sticky; it rinses away easily.)

Mix together the water and molasses, stirring well. To use: Soak your nails in the solution for 15–20 minutes or swab on clean nails in the evening before going to bed.

Yield: 2 ounces, enough for 1 nail soak for both hands

Zanzibar Foot Oil

1/4 cup light sesame oil or macadamia nut oil
5 drops clove oil

Off the east coast of Africa in the Indian Ocean lies Zanzibar. The island is famous for its lush and very fragrant spice plantations where cloves, cinnamon, and pepper are abundant. (Seventy-five percent of the world's cloves come from Zanzibar). This massage oil is especially well suited for foot massages because it contains clove oil, which is naturally antiseptic. Clove oil is available at many pharmacies, or you can make your own by soaking a few whole cloves in a tablespoon of oil overnight.

Mix together the two oils and pour into a clean container. To use: Massage a small amount into tired feet and legs.

Yield: 2 ounces

Pavlova Foot Treatment

Anna Pavlova was one of the world's best-loved ballerinas. Famous not just for her dancing, Pavlova was a great beauty who wore very little makeup. Her secret was plain white petroleum jelly, which she used on her entire body, especially her precious feet. I like to use this foot treatment in the evening before going to bed. I massage the rich jelly into my feet and then slip them into thick cotton socks—and wake up to smooth, soft skin.

¼ cup petroleum jelly
½ tablespoon vitamin E oil

Warm the petroleum jelly until it is just starting to melt. Stir in the vitamin E oil and mix well to blend. Allow the mixture to cool completely and spoon the cream into a clean container with a tight-fitting lid. To use: Massage a small amount into your feet and cover with clean socks.

Yield: 2½ ounces

Lincoln Footbath

1 teaspoon dried sage
1 teaspoon dried rosemary
10–12 juniper berries
5 whole cloves

President Abraham Lincoln was famous for saying, "When my feet hurt, I can't think." Footbaths were a favorite cure-all and much more common in Lincoln's time than they are now. A full bath was quite labor-intensive in those days because buckets of hot water first had to be heated and then carried to the bathtub. Try this spicy bath to revive your feet and mind.

Place all the ingredients in a cheesecloth square and tie securely or place them in a large tea ball. Fill a small tub with boiling water and place the dried bundle in the water. Let it steep until the water is cool enough for your feet. This can take 15–20 minutes. Then sit back and relax, allowing the fragrant water to soothe your feet. Pat your skin dry and massage a rich cream or natural oil into your feet.

Yield: ½ ounce, enough for 1 foot bath

Dream Pillow

*O*ne of the best cures for dark circles and dull skin is a good night's sleep. Rest is essential to our health and our skin, yet so many of us do not get enough! A Dream Pillow makes a welcome gift for people of all ages. You can stitch one up in one of many shapes and sizes using scraps of decorative fabrics embellished with a variety of notions. Slip one of these pretty scented cushions under your pillow, and you should dream for eight hours.

100 percent cotton or silk fabric
Dried lavender—soothing and relaxing
Dried mint—refreshing
Dried rosemary—strengthens your memory
Dried rose petals—calming
Flaxseeds or rice

With the right sides of fabric together, stitch a small pillowcase leaving one end open for filling. You may want to decorate your case with embroidery, buttons, tassels, or jewels. I like to make small patchwork pillows using fabric scraps.

Mix together enough rice or flaxseeds to loosely fill your pillow with one to two tablespoons of dried herbs. Add more herbs until the scent pleases you.

Fill the pillowcase with the herb mixture and stitch the open end closed.

To use: Shake the pillow gently to release the herbal scents. Place under your pillow or under your head and neck, and relax. Focus on the fragrance emitted from the Dream Pillow, and soon you will be fast asleep.

Yield: 1 pillow

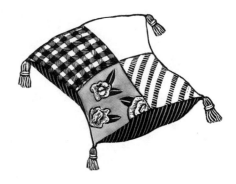

Neck Warmer

1 100 percent cotton bandanna
   scarf
2 pounds small-grain rice (I like to
   use pearl rice)

My husband often complains of a "stiff" neck. After a particularly painful one last winter, I sewed him this neck warmer. The design is very simple—a long cotton pillow stuffed with small-grain rice. You can heat the pillow in the microwave or clothes dryer, and the rice naturally retains the heat for up to an hour. I like to wear one while reading in bed on a cold winter night. It also makes a great après ski gift.

Fold the scarf on the diagonal. With right sides together, sew 1 long seam 4 inches from the fold. Trim ½ inch from sewing. Sew the ends together leaving a 1-inch opening in one end for filling.

Turn the pillow right side out. You should now have a long case 3 inches by 25 inches (approximately).

Using a funnel or paper cone, pour the rice into the pillow. Sew the open end shut.

To use: Heat in the microwave for 1 to 2 minutes. Check the temperature after 1 minute. Wrap around your neck and shoulders, and relax.

Note: You may also freeze the pillow for a cold treatment. This is a nice way to cool down in the summer heat. Keep the pillow dry. I prefer to store the pillows in plastic bags when not in use. The pillows can be reheated or refrozen for future use.

Yield: 1 pillow

Olive Oil Shaving Cream

It's a good policy for men to shower before they shave because the steam will soften their facial hair and make the process smoother and more comfortable. Moisturizing the hair is the most important thing a shaving cream can do. The addition of olive oil to this recipe creates a rich, moisturizing cream. Women may also enjoy using this recipe when shaving their legs.

¼ cup stearic acid powder
2 tablespoons extra-virgin olive oil
1 cup hot water
1 teaspoon borax
2 tablespoons grated soap

In a double boiler on the stove top, melt the stearic acid powder and oil until a clear liquid forms.

Mix together the hot water, borax, and soap, and stir until the borax and soap are completely dissolved. Pour the soap solution into a blender and blend well for about 1 minute. Slowly pour the melted stearic acid mixture into the soap solution. Blend on high until a smooth cream forms.

Pour into a clean container and allow to cool completely. To use, soften your beard with warm water and then apply the shaving cream to your face. Use a sharp, clean razor.

Yield: 8 ounces

Clark Gable Mustache Wax

Clark Gable was, for me, one of Hollywood's sexiest film legends. Like a lot of college women, I used to have a life-size poster of him on my dorm wall, posing as Rhett Butler from Gone with the Wind. *To this day I can see his warm smile and dark, well-groomed mustache. This recipe can also be used to groom unruly eyebrows and keep them in place.*

2 teaspoons grated beeswax
1 teaspoon castor oil

Mix together the beeswax and castor oil in a heat-resistant container. Heat the mixture gently in the microwave on High or on the stove top in a water bath, stirring continuously until the beeswax is melted.

Pour into a clean container and allow to cool until solid. To use: Rub your finger over the wax and apply sparingly to your mustache or eyebrows.

Yield: ½ ounce

Beauty Wreath

1 loofah sponge
Natural or colored raffia
1 small grapevine wreath
   (10–12 inches in diameter)
5 small bundles of dried herbs
3 small bottles of essential oil
   (your choice)
2 to 3 cinnamon sticks broken
   in half
5 dried star anise
Small beauty items: emery boards,
   nail brush, wooden combs,
   brushes, orange sticks, safety
   razors, pumice stone

This pretty wreath filled with useful beauty items is perfect for keeping in the bathroom. It makes a wonderful holiday gift since it provides a year's worth of pampering and beauty inspirations. Be creative and add to the wreath form any small beauty item that strikes your fancy.

Using a bread knife, slice the loofah sponge crosswise into ½-inch slices. Using the raffia, tie these round slices around the wreath. Tie all the items around the wreath until it looks full and the arrangement pleases you. Using several strands of raffia, make a large bow and attach it to the top of the wreath. You can tie small pieces of cinnamon stick and star anise onto the loose ends of the bow.

Yield: 1 wreath

Bay Leaf Bath Trees

Bay laurel comes to us from the Mediterranean. The leaves are aromatic and soothing. Dried laurel leaves added to the bath help relieve sore and aching muscles. Make a small topiary tree to place on your bathroom counter or give as a gift. To use, simply pick one or two of the leaves from your tree and add to your bathwater.

Florist clay or modeling clay
Small clay pot
1 large cinnamon stick
Natural moss or small rocks
1 small styrofoam cone
Straight pins
Dried bay leaves

Place a small amount of clay in the bottom of the clay pot and attach the cinnamon stick. Make sure that the cinnamon stick is above the pot edge. Fill the pot with moss or small rocks to hide the clay.

Gently slide the styrofoam cone over the cinnamon stick. You may want to make a hole first in the cone bottom. Starting from the bottom of the cone, pin one row of dried bay leaves around the cone. Continue pinning the leaves onto the cone, overlapping slightly so that the pinheads do not show.

Yield: 1 bath tree

Cinnamon Toothpaste

This is a spicy toothpaste that helps keep your teeth pearly white and your breath fresh. Baking soda neutralizes acids from plaque, helping to prevent gingivitis or gum disease, while the cinnamon gives the paste a great flavor! Don't forget to brush your gums and tongue, and rinse well. If the mixture seems a bit dry to you, add some more water.

2 teaspoons baking soda
1 teaspoon ground cinnamon
2 teaspoons water

Mix together all the ingredients to form a smooth paste using the back of a spoon. Use as you would any toothpaste and rinse well.

Yield: 1 ounce

Tooth Powders

Here are three basic tooth powders from Natural Beauty at Home. *They are very inexpensive and as effective as brand names. Make sure to replace your toothbrush as soon as the bristles start to wear out and keep your brush clean and dry between uses. Once a week I place mine in the dishwasher! Try to brush your teeth for at least two full minutes; placing an egg timer next to the bathroom sink is a simple way to keep track of the time. And remember the three most important things you can do for your teeth and gums: floss, floss, and floss! Even the best toothbrush cannot remove plaque under the gums and between the teeth.*

Classic: Baking soda is the classic tooth powder because it is a mild abrasive and is very effective at cleaning between the teeth and gums. Dip a damp toothbrush in a dish of baking soda and massage your teeth and gums.

Dried sage: Sage is a natural tooth whitener. It can be used alone or mixed with baking soda.

Citrus peels: Dried citrus peels finely ground in a coffee or spice grinder make a good tooth powder that is cleansing and has a mild citrus flavor. Use only the colored part, or zest, of the peel.

Tea Tree Oil Mouthwash

Tea tree oil from Australia is a natural antiseptic. As a mouthwash it helps keep your mouth hygienic and your breath fresh. It's also effective in preventing gum disease and kills germs that can cause tooth plaque. A clean, healthy mouth enhances your own natural beauty and self-confidence. Tea tree oil has a mild minty taste and a fragrance similar to eucalyptus. It can be found in many natural food stores and some pharmacies.

2 cups water
⅛ teaspoon tea tree oil
1 teaspoon aloe vera gel
1 vitamin C tablet, crushed
2 drops essential oil of peppermint
  or spearmint

Mix together all ingredients and stir well to blend. Pour into a clean container. To use: Rinse your mouth with approximately 1 teaspoon of mouthwash.

Yield: 16 ounces

Simple Clove Mouthwash

2 tablespoons whole cloves
2 cups boiling water

This is a simple mouthwash with a spicy taste. It will leave your whole mouth feeling fresh, and it's as easy to make as a cup of tea. Clove buds are easily found in the spice section of your local grocery store. They work well in this recipe because of their strong antiseptic properties.

Place the cloves in a heat-resistant container and cover with boiling water. Cover the container and let the mixture sit until cool. Strain the mouthwash and pour into a clean container. To use: Rinse your mouth with 1 teaspoon of the mouthwash.

Yield: 16 ounces

NEW YEAR HEAD-TO-TOE BEAUTY PARTY

"Ring out the old and ring in the new." A fun way to start the new year off right is with a head-to-toe beauty party.

This is sort of a grown-up slumber party (without staying up all night or having a séance). Book a popular local hairstylist for an at-home group appointment, and you can all start the year off with a new look and attitude.

Make your party announcements in the form of an appointment card, like those used by top salons. Say you will call to confirm their makeover. You can also print the party details on small mirrors or pocket calendars. Ask each guest to wear exercise or casual clothes.

(continued)

Borrow an instant camera and take "before" pictures as your guests arrive; these can be used as place cards and later given as a party favor along with their "after" photo. Start your party off with some yoga or stretching exercises, or go for a walk. You may also want everyone to meet at a local gym or aerobics class.

After the exercise session, get to work on your skin and hair. Mix up some facial masks and then give each other a manicure as the masks rest. You can also practice new hairstyles on each other—try a braid, chignon, or a dramatic French twist. There are even instructional videos you can rent and watch together.

Serve a healthy lunch or snack and talk about the new year ahead.

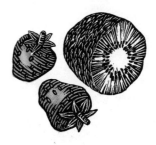

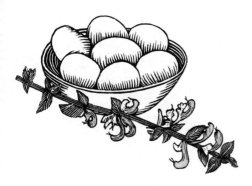

MERRY CHRISTMAS BASKET

For a wonderful way to pamper someone special this holiday season make up a basket filled with yuletide beauty and bath products. It will keep that special person looking and feeling her holiday best!

Suggested items to include:

Eggnog Lotion (page 49)
Foaming Vanilla Honey Bath (page 120)
Holiday washcloths
Candy Cane Bath Salts (page 59)
Pine Toner (page 45)
Fluffy cotton balls

Fill a natural-colored basket with fresh holiday greenery and tuck your gift items in among the fragrant boughs. Holiday washcloths are easy to make. Simply embroider a holiday design onto one corner; it's even easier to use fabric paint. Small items such as nail brushes, essential oils, or massage tools can be tied around the handles of your basket, and include a few jingle bells and candy canes for fun.

HAPPY HANUKKAH BASKET

Create a basket for a special family or friend to help celebrate the festival of lights. Bath items can be enjoyed by people of all ages and are perfect small presents for Hanukkah.

Suggested items to include:

Mashed Potato Hand Cream (page 203)
Dreidel
Rose Hip Skin Tonic (page 199)
Natural oils
Chocolate coins
Foaming Bath Salts
(in blue and white, page 225)

Find a pretty cardboard box and decorate the outside. Line the box with gold metallic paper or fabric and wrap each item in blue-and-white tissue paper. Don't forget to include plenty of gold coins (chocolate, of course) to be used for *gelt* when playing dreidel.

Spring Skin and Hair Care

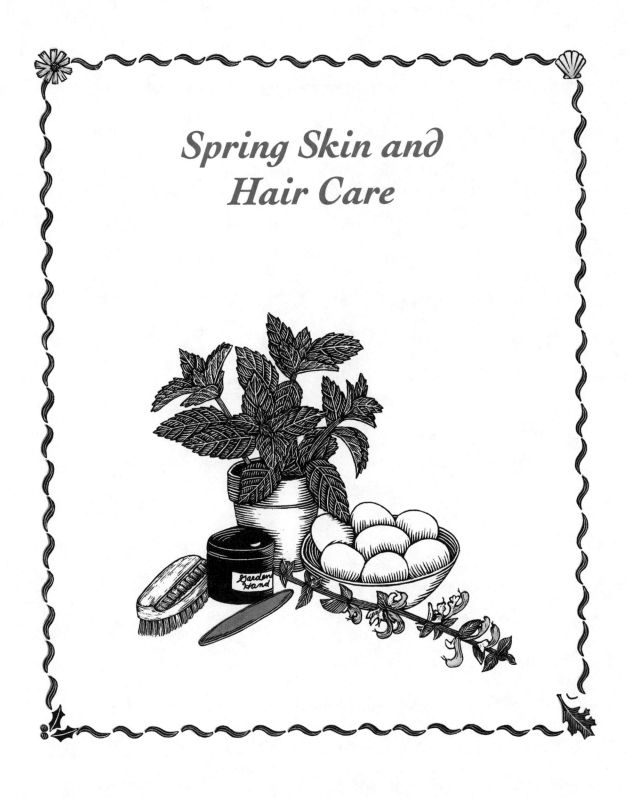

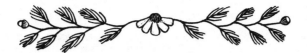

Spring is the season of renewal and celebration. The world is once again fragrant and green, the days are milder, and even the occasional rain shower is welcome because it helps the plants and flowers flourish. When I see fresh rhubarb in the market, I know spring is truly here! Lettuce, carrots, herbs, and eggs are some of my favorite ingredients to use this time of year in creating beauty products.

"Spring fever" is easy to catch, and I find myself spending as much time as I can spare outdoors in the yard. After a long winter spent studying garden books and seed catalogs, I am ready to get my hands dirty. I like to plant a small herbal beauty garden each year (see page 92). Herbs are some of the easiest plants to grow; some varieties, like mint, actually *thrive* when ignored! Herbs don't require a large amount of space and can be cultivated in a large container or window box. If you live in the city where a garden may be unheard of, plant your herbs in small terra-cotta pots indoors. Start an "herb exchange" with a few friends, each taking responsibility for a few varieties. You can then get together and have a garden beauty party creating bath vinegars, aromatic bath bundles, and herbal shampoos and rinses to take home and use. This is a great way to celebrate Earth Day in April.

Remember when you're outdoors to always use a good sunscreen. I like to wear a cotton scarf around my neck and a wide-brimmed hat to protect my skin from the sun. Also, garden gloves are a must! Scratch a bar of soap before putting on your gloves to keep your nails clean and supported. When working, don't forget to take breaks to smell the flowers. Pick a leaf or flower bud and take a minute to really focus on the scent. Learning to relax and take healthy breaks will increase your energy level, and you'll find you're more productive in the long run.

Vacations or "spring flings" are fun to plan during this time of year. If you are traveling by airplane through several time zones, you may want to try some aromatherapy cures for jet lag (see page 135) so you can avoid the fatigue brought on by travel. I have also included some ideas to try after you have arrived; see Hotel Room Beauty on page 136.

Spring is also a time of great festivity and joy. Weddings, graduations, and reunions are all popular springtime events. Looking and feeling your best is important and helps to nourish your self-esteem.

There are also many lovely gift ideas for this season. Pamper your mother with a special bath basket for Mother's Day in May or create a present for Dad on his special day in June. Wedding shower gifts for the bath are always fun to give. Include some pretty bath oil you've made, together with a set of new cotton towels. I love to give fresh flowers when possible with my gifts. They are always a welcome sight and give an instant boost! Create a special floral bouquet that can be admired and then diffused into a warm bath for a luxurious and sensual spring bathing experience.

For a description of common spring ingredients and where to find them, see page 18.

PLANT YOUR OWN BEAUTY GARDEN

The following is a list of some of my favorite herbs and vegetables that I plant in my garden each spring. You may want to try some of them. This is not a complete list, so please feel free to include your own personal preferences. There are many mail-order sources that specialize in new and unusual plants and seeds. Many of these plants are perennial, so they should come back for several years without replanting. They can also be grown in containers indoors.

HERBS

Basil: This is a popular and useful herb and comes in a variety of scents. Last year I planted cinnamon, lemon, and purple basil. Plant this annual in full sun and pinch back the flowers when they appear. The scent of basil is believed to be a natural aphrodisiac, and dried basil added to light vegetable oil makes a wonderful massage oil.

Calendula: Also known as "pot marigolds," these bright, annual orange and yellow flowers are cheery and dependable bloomers. Plant in full sun to partial shade. They will grow to a height of one to two feet. The flower petals can be dried and used in bath vinegars and hair rinses for highlighting red and blond hair.

Chamomile: A perennial low-growing lacy plant with daisylike flowers. Plant in full sun to partial shade. Dries easily, but cover with cheesecloth while drying to keep insects away from flowers. Makes wonderful herbal teas and fragrant baths.

Clary sage: A perennial that will grow to a height of 2–5 feet. Loves full sun, and flowers from June to July. After the first year, pale blue and lavender blossoms appear. Can be used fresh or dried. Clary sage is extremely aromatic and makes a good highlighting hair rinse for brunettes.

Lavender: A perennial flowering shrub that will grow 2–3 feet in height. Plant in full sun. Seeds come in white, pink, and purple varieties with slender gray-green leaves. Flowers from June to July and dries very easily for winter use. Lavender has a wonderful relaxing scent and a multitude of beauty uses.

Mint: Mint is my favorite herb to grow because it thrives even when ignored and comes in a wide variety of scents. I currently have several growing around my yard, including orange, eau de cologne, lavender, chocolate, peppermint, and spearmint. These plants grow in most locations and can be planted in full sun or partial shade. Mint spreads rampantly, so if you don't want your garden invaded with mint, plant it in a container. This herb loves to be cut frequently, and I use it in everything from perfumes and baths to scented drinks. Mint dries easily—simply hang in bunches to dry and store in airtight containers.

Rosemary: The scent of rosemary is believed to help improve your memory. It is a garden perennial that also does quite well indoors and can be grown as a garden topiary for fun. Plant in full sun to partial shade. It can be used fresh or dried. Rosemary-scented oil makes an excellent scalp treatment.

Parsley: Parsley is included in many gardens because it is easy to grow and has a number of practical uses. Plant the seeds in full sun to partial shade, and the parsley will grow up to 12 inches in height. This herb is an annual plant. We all know parsley is a powerful mouth deodorant, but it also has skin-softening properties and makes a soothing skin toner.

VEGETABLES

Cucumber: These plants like full sun and love to climb. They tend to dislike cold soil, so wait for three to four weeks after the last frost before planting them in the garden. Cucumber takes from forty-eight to seventy days to reach maturity. The classic cure for puffy eyes is cucumber slices placed over your eyelids. Cucumber juice can also be added to creams and lotions, and makes a soothing cure for a bad sunburn.

Loofah (Luffa) *sponges:* These relatives of the cucumber and gourd also love full sun and love to climb. Please see Growing Loofahs Sponges on page 97 for more information.

Tomatoes: Considered the queen of the garden, tomatoes are really very simple to grow. They love full sun and take fifty to ninety days to mature. Use wooden stakes or tomato cages to support the plants as they grow. Fresh tomatoes mixed with some yellow cornmeal make a good cleansing scrub for oily skin. They are mildly acidic, so sensitive skin types should use caution.

Gardener's Hand Cream

Gardening is especially hard on your hands—dry, rough hands with short nails are usually a good indicator of a beautiful garden. But this doesn't have to be the case. Massage just a small amount of this rich cream into your hands, making sure to dab some under each nail to condition them and keep out dirt. And always use garden gloves when possible; this alone will improve the condition of your hands. After cleaning up, use more of this cream to restore any lost moisture and to keep your hands soft and looking their best.

This hand cream is a great gift idea for any gardening friend. I like to package it in small terra-cotta pots (cover the hole with foil) and use a large cork—available at many hardware stores—for a lid. Use natural raffia to make a nice bow and include a new pair of garden gloves.

3 tablespoons grated beeswax
1 tablespoon liquid lanolin
1/2 cup light sesame oil (any light oil will work; I like sesame because it helps screen harmful ultraviolet rays from the sun)
2 tablespoons strong chamomile tea
1 tablespoon coconut oil
1 teaspoon honey
1/8 teaspoon baking soda

Combine all ingredients in a glass ovenproof container or double boiler. Heat in the microwave or over medium heat on the stove top until all the wax and oils are melted (do not boil), stirring well. Pour the melted mixture into a container or jar and allow to cool completely. Stir again when the mixture has cooled.

Yield: 4 ounces

Fizzing Bath Seeds

These effervescent bath salts are great fun to use and to give as a gift. First fill your tub up with warm water. Then throw in a scoop of these salts and watch them fizz and bubble. Add a few drops of your favorite essential oil and slip into the warm, soft water. Citric acid crystals, which are used in canning to keep fresh fruit from turning brown, can also be found in the vitamin section of your pharmacy.

1/3 cup baking soda
1/4 cup citric acid crystals or powder
1 tablespoon cornstarch

Mix together all the ingredients and place in a clean, dry container with a tight-fitting lid. Be careful to keep your salts dry because moisture will cause them to react and "fizz" in the container. To use: Sprinkle about ¼ cup of the salts into a warm tub of water.

Yield: 5 ounces, enough for 2 baths

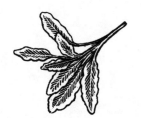

> ### *BEAUTY GARDEN KIT*
>
> In the spring I like to create beauty garden kits for my friends. I purchase a plain clay garden pot and decorate the outside with paints or glue pretty pictures around the rim. I fill the pot with seed packets, new garden gloves, a sturdy garden trowel, and a jar of Gardener's Hand Cream (see page 95) in an attractive plastic jar. This is everything they will need to create a beautiful garden full of herbs and flowers to enjoy all year long. If your friends live in the city where growing space can be hard to find, adapt your kit to herbs and flowers that can be planted in a large wood or clay container.

GROWING LOOFAH SPONGES

Many people are surprised to learn that the loofah (some spell it *luffa*) sponge they use in the bath actually comes from the garden and not the sea. The loofah belongs to a large family of plants that includes gourds, squashes, pumpkins, cucumbers, and melons. They are most closely related to cucumbers in appearance and growing habits. Loofahs are easy to grow and are a multipurpose vegetable. You can eat them or use them as scrubbers in the kitchen or as a beauty tool in the bath or shower.

Loofah seeds can be found in the seed section of many garden shops or may be ordered from mail-order catalogs that specialize in exotic vegetables.

TO GROW

Loofah seeds are easy to work with. They are large flat black seeds, much like watermelon seeds in appearance, so that even small children can easily plant them. Loofahs grow on vines and love to climb. They also love full sun, so choose a sunny location next to a fence or use a trellis. You can also grow loofahs in containers with tomato cages or a wire trellis.

Loofah plants are sensitive to the cold, so you may want to plant the seeds inside until all danger of frost is past. Use soil that is rich in organic material or humus. Plant the seeds ¾ inch to 1 inch deep and cover with another inch of compost or manure.

Water daily until the plants are established, then water deeply every seven days. Fertilize the vines when yellow flowers appear. The vegetable that will become the sponge is green, smooth, and resembles a large cucumber. Loofahs can reach 18 inches in length and weigh up to five pounds, and as many as twenty-five loofahs may grow on a single vine. Some people like to remove all of the first flowers from the vine because they feel this produces a higher quality of sponge.

TO HARVEST

Allow the loofahs to ripen on the vine until the skin turns dark yellow or brown. After picking, soak them in a bucket of water to soften the brown outer skin. Peel off all the brown skin, remove the seeds, and let dry. Store the seeds for next year's crop. After removing the peel and seeds, let the "skeletons" of the loofahs dry in the sun. These fibrous skeletons become your sponges.

To Use

Mature loofahs contain a netlike fibrous skeleton that resembles woven fabric. When wet, it is soft and pliable and very long-wearing. It also holds water like a sea sponge.

When used in the kitchen, loofah sponges are a gentle, nonscratching scrubber ideal for glassware and china. They are also good for cleaning vegetables, such as carrots and potatoes.

In the bath they are excellent exfoliators. Gently rubbing the loofah over wet skin removes dead skin cells and surface dirt. Using a loofah is also beneficial for your circulation and gives your skin a healthy glow.

You can make your own loofah soap by adding bits of the chopped sponge to melted soap. The following recipe is for a simple loofah soap that makes an excellent scrubbing bar for your body. They also make nice gifts tied up in pretty paper or fabric.

Loofah Soap

Petroleum jelly for greasing soap molds
1 bar bath soap, grated (approximately 1¼ cups)
1 tablespoon water
1 tablespoon finely chopped loofah sponge (use kitchen scissors to cut up)

Note: A simple rule of thumb when melting soap is to use only $\frac{1}{10}$ the amount of water as soap. For example, if you have 20 ounces of soap, you would use 2 ounces of water. An average bar of soap is 3½ to 5 ounces. I usually allow 1 tablespoon (½ ounce) per bar of soap.

Lightly grease the inside of the soap molds using the petroleum jelly. Place the soap and water into the top part of your double boiler or in an ovenproof dish in a saucepan of water and heat gently over medium heat, stirring occasionally. Heat until the soap is completely melted and resembles a smooth, fluffy white pudding. This may take up to 30 minutes. The soap starts out looking very dry and grainy, and then turns thick like pudding. Stir in the chopped loofah sponge and mix well.

It is important not to use direct heat, and do not allow the mixture to boil.

When all the soap is melted and smooth, carefully spoon the mixture into your prepared molds. It's okay if the molds overflow a bit because the soap may settle a bit; you can always trim away any excess after it has cooled. You will want to work quickly since the soap begins to cool immediately. Tap the edge of your molds gently to remove any air in the soap.

Allow the molds to sit until the soap is completely cool. Remove and place the soap shapes on a wire baking rack to dry. Let the soap sit for at least 24 hours; the longer the soap can sit, the better. If the soap seems a bit rough around the edges, you can smooth it with a sharp knife.

Yield: 1–2 bars of soap depending on mold size

SOAP MOLDS

Cookie cutters, muffin tins, and small cardboard boxes all make good soap molds. Basically any small container can be used. I prefer to use cookie cutters placed on top of a sheet of foil. When cool the soap shapes can simply be pushed out of the mold.

Loofah Vine Toner

2 tablespoons loofah vine water
1 tablespoon sake (rice wine)
2 tablespoons rosewater

Loofah vine water is used in Japan as a simple beauty lotion that protects and moisturizes the skin. Try this simple recipe to make an ideal toner for delicate skin. To extract the water from the vine, cut 12 inches of the vine and place the cut end upright in a clean jar or bottle. Let the cutting sit overnight until the sap or "water" has drained out into the container. Sake is a Japanese rice wine available at Asian markets and some grocery stores.

Mix together all the ingredients and stir well. Pour into a clean container with a tight-fitting lid. To use: Apply to the skin using a clean cotton ball.

Yield: 2½ ounces

Loofah Salt Glow

To enhance the effectiveness of your loofah sponge try this body scrub recipe. It will help keep your skin healthy and glowing by removing any dead, flaky skin and boosting your circulation. Please note that this treatment is intended for your body only; the scrub is too harsh for delicate facial skin.

¼ cup ground sea salt
1 loofah sponge

In the bath or shower, pat the sea salt onto damp skin and gently run the loofah sponge over your skin in a circular pattern. Pay particular attention to classic rough skin spots such as elbows, knees, and heels. Rinse well and follow with a rich body lotion.

Yield: 2 ounces, enough for 1 whole body treatment

Oatmeal and Almond Scrub

Oatmeal is a well-known and popular home beauty ingredient. It is especially well suited for individuals with sensitive skin because it is mild and soothing. Mixed together with ground almonds, this scrub can remove embedded dirt and help prevent blackheads. Old-fashioned whole oatmeal works best and is less expensive than the quick-cooking grains. I use my coffee grinder to finely grind the oats and almonds. You can also use a blender, food processor, or mortar and pestle.

¼ cup finely ground oatmeal
¼ cup finely ground almonds

Mix together the two ingredients and stir well. Place in a clean, dry container. To use: Place approximately 1 teaspoon of the scrub in the palm of your hand and add enough water to make a soft paste. Spread the mixture on your face and massage into the skin. Rinse well with warm water.

Yield: 4 ounces

Alfalfa Sprout Scrub

1 tablespoon fresh alfalfa sprouts
1 teaspoon rice flour or ground
   oatmeal (optional)

*A*lfalfa sprouts are available in most grocery stores in the produce section. They make a vitamin- and protein-rich cleansing scrub from which all skin types can benefit. They are also easy to grow at home. Use only organically grown seeds (available from health food stores and some garden supply houses). Wash ¼ cup of seeds, place in a bowl or jar, and cover with lukewarm water. Let stand overnight. Drain and rinse the seeds, and drain again thoroughly. Place the seeds in a large glass jar, cover the top with a piece of cheesecloth or nylon mesh, and secure tightly. Place the jar on its side, so that the seeds form a thin layer, in a dark place where it is warm and humid. Rinse the seeds at least three times every day by pouring lukewarm water into the jar, swirling it around, and draining it. You should begin to see sprouts develop in three to five days. When small green leaves appear, you may place the jar in direct sunlight. When they are about one inch long, store the sprouts in the refrigerator, where they will stay fresh for three to five days.

With kitchen scissors, cut the sprouts into small pieces. For a smoother, cleanserlike paste, mix in some rice flour or oatmeal and water. To use: Wash your face with the alfalfa sprouts and rinse well with cool water. This treatment can be used all over the body.

Yield: 1 ounce, enough for 1 treatment.

Lettuce Cleansing Lotion

Crisp, fresh lettuce makes a sublime facial lotion that is especially well suited to sensitive skin. This simple cleansing solution will also soothe burned or irritated skin. Lettuce contains vitamins, sulfur, silicon, and phosphorus—all important ingredients for maintaining a healthy complexion.

½ head of lettuce
4 cups water
⅛ teaspoon tincture of benzoin

Place the lettuce in a medium-size saucepan and cover with the water. Bring the water to a boil over medium heat. Lower the heat and simmer for 1 hour. Remove from the heat and allow the mixture to cool completely. Strain off all solids and stir in the tincture of benzoin. Pour into a clean container. Use this lotion to cleanse your skin.

Yield: 16 ounces

Graduation Scrub

Graduation is a time of great personal satisfaction, change, and celebration. It is also a time when you want to look your best. Make up a batch of this simple cleansing powder and use it to make your complexion glow. This recipe also makes a nice gift for the college bound. Include a small jar of the scrub along with other essentials and package inside a plastic bucket or tackle box.

¼ cup oatmeal
¼ cup sliced almonds
1 tablespoon cornstarch
1 tablespoon dried chamomile
    flowers

Place all the ingredients in a food processor or blender and finely grind into a powder. Pour into a clean, dry container. To use: Mix together 1–2 teaspoons in the palm of your hand with some water and work into a smooth paste. Use this mixture to cleanse your skin.

Yield: 6 ounces

COLLEGE-BOUND BASKET

Getting ready for college is an exciting and hectic time. A good gift for a graduating high school senior is a plastic bucket or tote filled with some healthy gifts and bath essentials. The bucket can be used to carry toiletries to and from the shower.

Suggested items to include:

Decorated Hair Accessories (page 218)

Scented Shower Gels
(see April Showers gels on page 116)

Loofah sponge

Scented Dusting Powder (page 224)

Florida Grapefruit Freshener (page 46)

New toothbrush

Eye Rest Pillow (page 130)

Fill a plastic tackle box or brightly colored bucket with shower essentials. Personalize the box and gift so they don't get lost. I like to use acrylic paint pens that work on a variety of surfaces and come in many colors. Write funny notes and messages on each item. For example "Smile" on the toothbrush or "You are beautiful!" on a new hairbrush. These small everyday reminders of your love and support will be appreciated, especially during those first few months away from home.

Lilac Skin Toner

Lilacs are one of my favorite spring flowers. The moment they begin to bloom I fill our house with bouquets of these fragrant, old-fashioned blossoms. This is a recipe for a gentle toner made from the green leaves of the lilac bush. The leaves add a wonderful fragrance to this toner and have mild skin-cleansing properties. It is good for all skin types, especially sensitive skin.

1 cup boiling water
½ cup freshly picked lilac leaves

Pour the water over the leaves and let the mixture cool completely. Strain off the leaves and pour into a clean bottle. To use: Apply to your skin with a clean cotton ball.

Yield: 8 ounces

Parsley Skin Freshener

We all know parsley is a powerful mouth freshener, but it also makes a mild and gentle toner for the skin. Use this freshener throughout the day to keep your complexion clean and radiant. Parsley is easy to find in any grocery or vegetable market. It's also a snap to grow in your herb garden, whether in your yard or on your windowsill.

½ cup chopped parsley
1 cup boiling water

Place the parsley in a ceramic bowl and pour the boiling water over the herb. Allow the mixture to cool completely, then strain and pour into a clean container. To use: Apply to the skin using a clean cotton ball.

Yield: 8 ounces

Queen Isabella Sherry Toner

3 tablespoons distilled water
2 tablespoons rosewater
2 tablespoons sherry wine

During the fifteenth century, Queen Isabella ruled the Spanish kingdom of Castile and Aragon with her husband, King Ferdinand. The queen was very supportive of Christopher Columbus's quest to find the Indies by sailing west, which resulted in the discovery of America in 1492. Today, April 22 is celebrated as Queen Isabella Day in Spain. This recipe contains sherry—an amber-colored, fortified wine from the Castilian and Aragon regions of Spain. The sherry also makes a mildly astringent toner that has clarifying, skin-enhancing properties.

Mix all the ingredients together. Bottle in an airtight container. To use: Apply to your skin using a clean cotton ball.

Yield: 3½ ounces

Mint Julep Toner

½ cup rosewater
½ teaspoon granulated sugar
2 tablespoons Kentucky bourbon
1 tablespoon dried mint leaves

The Kentucky Derby is the oldest continuously run horse race in the United States. It is held each year on the first Saturday of May at Churchill Downs in Louisville, Kentucky. Millions worldwide watch the "run for the roses"—so-called because a blanket of roses is presented to the winning horse and jockey. Mint juleps are the beverage of choice at this exhilarating event. Try this recipe not just in May but year-round for a refreshing start to your day.

Mix together all the ingredients, cover, and let sit overnight. Filter the liquid and pour into a clean container. (I use a coffee filter fitted inside a kitchen funnel.) Pour the liquid into a clean container with a tight-fitting lid. To use: Apply to your skin using a clean cotton ball.

Yield: 5 ounces

Green Tea Skin Toner

Green tea was brought to Japan by monks returning from their studies at the great Zen monasteries of twelfth-century China. At that time green tea functioned as an aid to meditation and health. Today, it is one of the most widely used nonalcoholic beverages in the world. It is also an excellent skin toner because it contains antioxidants such as vitamins C and E which help to strengthen your skin's natural defenses. This toner works especially well as an anti-irritant and can be used to soothe aggravated skin and sunburn.

½ cup pure spring water
2 teaspoons green tea leaves

Bring the water to a boil. Place the tea leaves in a clean glass or ceramic bowl. Pour the boiling water over the leaves and allow them to steep for 2–3 minutes. Strain the tea leaves and allow the liquid to cool. To use: Apply to the face with cotton or gauze. Do not rinse off.

Yield: 4 ounces

Gentle Eye Makeup Remover

Castor oil is excellent for removing eye makeup. I like to use this combination of castor, canola, and olive oils to remove my mascara in the evening. Even the most stubborn makeup glides off effortlessly with this light oil mixture.

1 tablespoon canola oil
1 tablespoon castor oil
1 tablespoon light olive oil

Mix together the three oils and pour into a clean container. To use: Pour a small amount of oil onto a clean cotton pad and gently wipe over your upper and lower eyelashes and eyelids.

Yield: 1½ ounces

Elbow Grease

¼ cup grated cocoa butter
2 tablespoons sesame oil
1 tablespoon avocado oil
1 tablespoon grated beeswax

If you have dry, rough skin but long for it to be soft and smooth, you need to apply a little "elbow grease" to your body. This oil-rich ointment can be used anywhere you need a little extra moisturizing effort.

Combine all the ingredients in an ovenproof glass container. Place the container with the mixture in a water bath or in the microwave and gently heat the contents until the cocoa butter and beeswax are melted. Pour the melted mixture into a clean jar and allow it to cool completely. Stir the cooled mixture.

Yield: 4 ounces

Gaia (Mother Earth) Clay Mask Collection

2 tablespoons clay
1–2 tablespoons spring water

Gaia is the Greek name for Mother Earth. Earthen clay is one of the oldest natural beauty treatments; it has been used to deep-cleanse the skin for centuries. The effects are immediate! After just a ten-minute facial, you will have tighter pores and more radiant skin. The clay draws oils from your pores and helps rid your skin of any surface dirt and dead skin cells. Natural clay's absorbent properties and wealth of minerals make for excellent face and body masks. The natural clays you can purchase come from purified earth, and their colors are derived from the minerals they contain. It is important for cosmetic use to use clay that has been purified. The soil from your garden will not do; it contains levels of bacteria that could be more harmful than helpful. Natural food stores and pharmacies are a good source of natural clays. Clays are also used in dry shampoos, in hair conditioners, and as thickeners in some cream recipes.

Fuller's earth: A fine gray clay powder that comes from algae found on sea- and riverbeds and is particularly high in magnesium silicate. The name comes from its use in making woolen fabrics. "Fulling" was a way of increasing the weight and bulk of the cloth by shrinking and beating it; a fuller was a person who made the woolen material.

Kaolin clay: Sometimes called China clay, this is a fine white powder originally obtained from Kaoling Hill in Kiangsi Province in southeast China. Kaolin clay is rich in aluminum silicate and is also used in the manufacturing of fine porcelain. This white clay will swell in water and makes a good thickening ingredient for facial masks and creams.

French green clay: A fine, pale green clay that comes from a quarry in southern France. It is rich in magnesium, dolomite, and silica, and is a highly absorbent clay. It may also be used as a deodorizer and cleanser. French green clay mixes very easily with water because it contains no sand or quartz.

Bentonite: A white clay found in the midwestern United States and Canada. It is high in aluminum silicate, magnesium, and iron. Bentonite is highly absorbent and can hold up to fifteen times its own volume of water or oil.

Rhassoul mud: Rhassoul is a natural clay or mud from the Atlas mountain range that runs parallel to the Mediterranean coast through Morocco, northern Algeria, and Tunisia. This clay is an effective cleanser and works well on oily hair. It can be found at natural food stores.

Mix the clay together with a little water until you have a smooth paste. Apply to your skin with fingertips and leave on for 15 minutes. Rinse with warm water and pat dry.

Variations:

OILY SKIN: Add ½ tablespoon lemon juice or apple cider vinegar.

NORMAL SKIN: Use milk or yogurt in place of spring water.

DRY SKIN: Add ½ tablespoon light oil.

Yield: 1 ounce, enough for 1 facial treatment

Body Mud Pack

½ cup powdered clay—your choice (see page 109)
¼ cup spring water

Playing in the mud when you were a child was pure bliss. Many spas today swear by their mineral-rich clay content for deep skin cleansing and gentle exfoliation. This treatment is a bit messy but the effect is immediate, and your skin will be glowing when you are done. Make sure to follow up with a moisturizer because the mud can dry out some skin types.

Mix together the clay and water to form a smooth paste. You may need to add a bit more clay or water; you want the paste to have a puddinglike consistency. Spread the mud evenly over your face and body, using a medium-size paintbrush or spatula. If you do not want to cover the whole body, just apply to your torso and arms. Wrap up in a large towel or old robe to keep

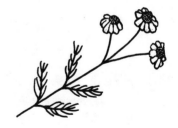

HAPPY EARTH DAY

Earth Day began in 1970 as a response to a suggestion made by Wisconsin senator Gaylord Nelson. Nelson thought a day should be set aside for serious discussion of environmental issues. More than one thousand cities and towns held a "Save the Earth" day on April 22, 1970. Today, Earth Day has become an annual celebration and educational exploration of green issues in more than 140 countries worldwide. Gather your friends together and celebrate Earth Day this year. Plan a trip to your local recycling center; clean up a park, beach, or your own neighborhood. Afterward, invite everyone over to plant individual beauty gardens in clay pots using small herb plants or seeds, or create some of the products in this book for sharing with your community.

Keep the world beautiful!

warm while you allow the mud to dry. After 15 to 20 minutes, shower with warm water followed by a rinse of the coolest water you can stand. Pat your skin dry with a towel and moisturize well.

Yield: 4 ounces, enough for 1 whole body treatment

Carrot Buttermilk Mask

2 tablespoons fresh carrot juice
2 tablespoons powdered buttermilk

This is an ideal facial mask for normal to oily skin types. (If you have dry skin, add 1 teaspoon of light oil to the mixture.) Carrot juice is rich in vitamin A—the "beauty" vitamin, so important for healthy skin and hair. You may purchase fresh carrot juice or make your own. Buttermilk is a natural astringent and cleanser full of calcium and protein.

Mix together the carrot juice and buttermilk into a smooth paste. Spread the mixture over clean skin and leave on for 10–15 minutes. Rinse well with tepid water and pat your skin dry.

Yield: 1 ounce, enough for 1 facial mask

Egg Masks

The classic facial, an egg mask, has been used by women for centuries. It consists simply of a raw egg spread on the face and left to dry, then rinsed off with cool water. My grandmother used this simple mask once a week to keep her skin youthful and glowing. Here are a few variations on this at-home beauty staple.

Egg mask for dry skin: Mix together 1 raw egg and 1 tablespoon of honey. Spread on your face and neck, and let sit for 15–20 minutes. Rinse well with tepid water.

Egg mask for oily skin: Mix together 1 egg white and 1 tablespoon of oatmeal. Spread on your face and neck, and let sit for 15–20 minutes. Rinse well with tepid water. This mask is good for removing blackheads.

Egg mask for normal skin: Mix together 1 egg and 1 teaspoon of fresh sour cream. Sour cream is rich in lactic acid and helps soften and remove surface impurities and dead skin cells, leaving your skin soft and smooth. Spread on your face and neck, and let sit for 15–20 minutes. Rinse well with tepid water.

Yield: 1–2 ounces, enough for 1 facial mask

Miss Muffett Mask

1 teaspoon powdered whey
½ teaspoon rosewater
1 teaspoon honey

Dr. Thomas Muffett, an entomologist who lived during the sixteenth century in England, wrote a brief and charming rhyme for his daughter Patience and in the process paid eternal homage to English culinary habits. This now-famous rhyme has done as much for "curds and whey" as it has for spiders! Whey, which is a by-product of cheese-making, is the key ingredient in this complexion conditioner. It makes an excellent source of protein. I purchase powdered dairy whey at my local health food store.

Combine the whey powder and rosewater, and stir well. Add the honey and continue stirring until the mixture is well blended. Spread the creamy lotion onto a clean face and neck, and let sit for 30 minutes. Rinse with warm water followed by cool.

Yield: 1 ounce, enough for 1 facial mask

Silk Facial Mask

1 piece of silk 10 inches square
Face pattern — use the one on page
    247 or make your own
2 tablespoons facial toner or fruit
    juice

By using a thin natural fabric such as silk or cotton cheese-cloth, it's easy to transform selected facial toners or fruit juices into refreshing facial masks. These pretty cloth masks can be reused as long as they are cleaned with a mild soap and left to air-dry thoroughly. I like to use old silk scarves, but any thin, clingy, natural fabric will do.

Place your facial mask pattern over the silk pattern and trace around the outline. Cut out the mask.

To use: Pour approximately 2 tablespoons of liquid (toner or fruit juice) into a shallow dish. Place the cloth mask into the dish and allow the liquid to be absorbed by the fabric. Place the damp cloth over your face and leave on for 15–20 minutes. (You may want to lie down to keep the cloth in place.) Remove the cloth, rinse your face well, and pat your skin dry.

Fruit juice suggestions:

NORMAL TO DRY SKIN TYPES: apple, pear, peach, raspberry, grape.

OILY SKIN TYPES: tomato, white grape, diluted lemon juice or grapefruit juice (1 tablespoon to ½ cup water).

Note: This mask can also be used with your favorite astringent in place of the toner or fruit juice.

Yield: 1 facial mask

Flower Petal Steam Facial

Spring is the season for flowers. After a colorless winter, the world seems fragrant and in full bloom. Gather a bouquet of spring flowers for your home, and just before they fade, use the soft petals to create this gentle facial steam to keep your skin soft. In this recipe I like to use a combination of lilac, rose, camellia, pansy, and primrose petals. (Note: I would use only edible flowers in this recipe, as all of these listed are.)

2 cups water
½ cup fresh flower petals

Bring the water to a boil, remove from the heat, add the flower petals, and stir. Let the mixture sit for 5 minutes. Lean over the pot, at least 12 inches from the surface, and drape a towel over your head to form a tent. Close your eyes and let the steam rise over your face for 5 minutes. Rinse with cool water and pat dry.

Yield: 16 ounces, enough for 1 facial steam treatment

April
Showers

½ cup liquid soap
1 teaspoon almond or sesame oil
4 drops essential oil (see chart
   below for ideas)

*S*howers and shower gels are more popular today than ever. I love to make my own scented shower gels—they're so simple to create. I buy plain unscented liquid soap by the gallon and transform it into dozens of unique shower gels using my scented oils. My favorite for early-morning showers is two drops of essential oil of lavender and two drops of essential oil of rosemary. These, incidentally, make delightful quick gifts. Pour the finished products into small plastic water bottles with the pull-out "sports"-style caps and tie a big bow around the neck using plastic weatherproof ribbon.

Mix together all ingredients and stir well. Pour into a clean plastic container (safer than glass in the shower).

SUGGESTED SHOWER GEL SCENTS

Relaxing: Choose one or a combination of two or three:
   Chamomile
   Neroli
   Rose
   Lavender
   Ylang-ylang

Energizing: Choose one or a combination of two or three:
   Bergamot
   Geranium
   Juniper
   Eucalyptus
   Rosemary
   Lemongrass

Yield: 4 ounces

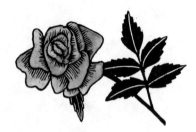

Rose Bouquet Bath

Nothing seems more indulgent than a bath strewn with gorgeous rose petals. If you're fortunate enough to receive a beautiful bouquet of fragrant roses, just before the blooms fade, carry them into the bathroom and cast their petals into your bath. Or venture out into the garden and pick the petals off the heads of roses in full bloom. (They will drop to the ground in a few days.) The scent of rose petals is said to banish melancholy. Their astringent quality will help cleanse and tone the skin.

Several large handfuls of fresh rose petals, approximately 2 cups

Fill the bath with warm water (not too hot). Cast the fresh petals over the water. You may also use a drop or two of rose oil. Slip into the warm water and relax.

Yield: 1 bath

Aromatic Bath Bundles

The scents from these little bundles can create certain moods or mental states. The scent of peppermint, for example, can be very energizing. The use of scents and aromatic ingredients is called Aromatherapy. Tie up some fresh herbs and flowers inside squares of muslin or cheesecloth and hang the bundle under the bath spout when filling your tub. You may also want to include some oatmeal or barley to help soften the water. When giving these as gifts, I use dried herbs and flowers and place three to five bundles inside a pretty jar or cellophane bag. Enjoy the sweet fragrance these herbs bring to your bath.

*½ cup fresh herbs and flowers or
  ¼ cup dried herbs and flowers for
  each bath
1–2 tablespoons oatmeal or barley
  (optional)*

Selection of herbs:

INVIGORATING: rosemary, sage, and thyme

RELAXING: chamomile and lavender

SOOTHING: chamomile and mint

Place the herbs and flowers in the middle of a large square of cheesecloth or muslin. Gather up the ends and tie with a length of cotton string; make sure the string is long enough to hang from the bath faucet. To use: Hang the bath bundle under the bath faucet when filling the tub with warm water. While bathing, you may remove the sack and rub it over your skin as a gentle cleanser.

Yield: One 2–4-ounce bath bundle, enough for 1 bath

Scented Milk Bath

2 cups dried powdered milk
1 tablespoon dried orange peel
2 teaspoons dried lavender flowers
2 teaspoons dried rosemary

Fresh milk has been used as a skin beautifier for centuries. It is high in protein, calcium, and vitamins, and is easily absorbed by the skin, leaving it soft and radiant. This recipe uses dry powdered milk scented with dried herbs and citrus peels to create a creamy, indulgent bath. Bathing in milk is still a classic beauty ritual. Use old glass milk bottles as interesting containers for your milk bath mixtures.

Mix together all the ingredients and pour into a clean milk bottle or container. To use: Pour ½ cup of the milk bath mixture into a warm bath and stir through the water. Soak in the tub for 20 minutes.

Yield: 16 ounces, enough for 4 baths

MOTHER'S DAY BASKET

All mothers are beautiful and special, but how often we take them for granted! Make up a beauty basket that will pamper and please your mother; fill it with her favorite scents and colors. Traditionally, mothers are served breakfast in bed on this day. This year let her start off with a long, warm bath followed by that breakfast.

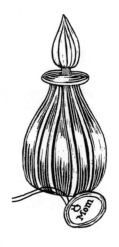

Suggested items to include:

Scented Dusting Powder (page 224)
Foaming Vanilla Honey Bath (page 120)
Eye Rest Pillow (page 130)
DO NOT DISTURB sign for the bathroom
Fizzing Bath Seeds (page 95)
Flower Power Cologne (page 130)

Personalize grosgrain ribbon with children's names using fabric or permanent felt tip markers. Use the ribbon to tie up your gift. Photocopy a favorite photo and paste it onto the front of a homemade card, and put a note or poem inside telling your mother how special she is.

Foaming Vanilla Honey Bath

1 cup oil
½ cup honey
½ cup liquid soap
1 tablespoon vanilla extract

Adding honey to the bath makes your skin feel silky smooth. It is one of my favorite beauty recipes because of its simplicity and effectiveness. This foaming bath uses golden honey and vanilla to create a delicious, subtle scent. Made from kitchen basics, this rich bath is full of fragrant, foaming bubbles. For a special gift, I like to package the bath liquid in multicolored glass bottles. Use silicone glue and attach a few glass marbles or beads to an ordinary cork for an interesting bottle stopper.

Mix together all the ingredients and pour into a clean bottle with a tight-fitting stopper or lid. To use: Shake before using. Pour ¼ cup into the bathtub under running water.

Yield: 16 ounces, enough for 8 baths

Stress Therapy Balls

½ cup white millet birdseed or
  any fine-grain birdseed
  (no sunflower seeds)
1 small plastic sandwich bag
Tape
Scissors
3 latex balloons, 9-inch size (I like
  to use a variety of bright colors)

These balls are quite easy to make and fun to give. I have seen them sold in beauty boutiques for up to $10 each! Stress therapy balls are a desk set essential for a busy executive because they soothe and release tension with every squeeze of the hand. Give one to your overworked accountant this tax season. If you package them in groups of three, they can even be used as juggling balls—and are generally considered an excellent hand exercise tool. This is also a good project for children. I have a basketful of these colorful balls at my house, and visitors young and old love to play with them!

Pour the birdseed into the plastic bag, twist to close, and tape down the twisted end. You will have a small round package. Cut the long stem end off the 3 balloons. Stretch the first balloon around the plastic bag to cover it. Stretch the second balloon over the first balloon, making sure to cover the cut end of the first balloon.

If you like, you can make small decorative slits or cuts in the last balloon. These will allow the colors of the balloon underneath to show through. Stretch this last balloon over the other two. You now have a colorful ball to have fun with.

Yield: 1 ball

Clay Hair Mask

Natural clays also function as deep conditioners for your hair and scalp. The clay cleanses the pores on your scalp, which is especially beneficial for oily skin and helps prevent dandruff. The amount of clay needed may vary depending on the length of your hair. This recipe is designed for shoulder-length hair.

¼ cup powdered clay (I like Rhassoul mud or French green clay)
2 tablespoons mineral water
½ teaspoon cider vinegar (optional)

Mix the water, clay, and vinegar together into a smooth paste. Massage into your scalp and hair (you may also use on your face). Leave the mask on for 10–15 minutes, then rinse well with warm water — no soap — and dry gently with a soft towel. You may need to rinse the hair for several minutes to remove all the clay.

Yield: 2 ounces, enough for 1 treatment

Indian Champo (Shampoo)

¼ cup honey or light corn syrup
½ cup glycerin
1 tablespoon witch hazel
¼ cup orange flower water
2 tablespoons bee pollen (optional)
1 teaspoon liquid soap
1 tablespoon vodka

In 1870, British hairdressers coined the word shampoo *from the Hindu word* Champo *which means "to massage" or "to knead." (The British government had just taken control of India, and using Hindu phrases was considered very fashionable.) A shampoo was available only to patrons of the most chic British salons. Use this recipe to give yourself a thorough, soapy scalp massage that will improve your scalp's circulation and the overall appearance of your hair. Because this recipe contains bee pollen and honey, it may lighten dark hair. If you have dark hair, you can replace the honey with light corn syrup and leave out the bee pollen.*

Combine all the ingredients and shake well to mix. Use as you would any shampoo product.

Yield: 8 ounces

Natural Highlighting Shampoo

½ cup water
⅓ cup fresh chamomile, lavender, or rosemary
½ cup mild shampoo or liquid castile soap
2 tablespoons glycerin

Certain herbs added to your favorite shampoo can bring out your hair's natural highlights. Chamomile makes a mild shampoo that is perfect for fine light-colored hair; these flowers have a mild bleaching effect. If you have dark hair, I would suggest using rosemary or lavender to enhance your natural color.

Mix together the water and herbs, and heat gently to make a strong infusion, or tea. Let the mixture steep for at least 20 minutes, then strain. Add the shampoo and glycerin to the herbal water and stir well.

Pour the shampoo into a clean plastic bottle and let the mixture sit overnight to thicken.

To use: Shampoo as you would normally and rinse well.

Yield: 8 ounces

Rhubarb Hair Rinse

Rhubarb is a great green leafy plant with pink and red stems, or stalks. These stalks are what you see for sale at the produce stand, and they make a wonderful hair-lightening rinse. Simmered in white wine or water the rhubarb will lighten your hair considerably. Regular use of this rinse will cause dramatic golden highlights in your hair.

3 fresh rhubarb stalks
2 cups white wine or water

Chop the rhubarb into small pieces and place in a medium-size saucepan. Cover with the wine or water and simmer for 30 minutes. Remove from the heat and let the mixture sit for another 30 minutes, then strain the liquid. Use the liquid as a hair rinse or mix together with 1–2 tablespoons of white kaolin clay to form a paste.

To use: Leave the mixture on clean, damp hair for 20 minutes to an hour, depending on the degree of lightening desired. I would suggest starting with 20 minutes and then increasing the time spent with the next treatment.

Yield: 12 ounces, enough for 1 to 2 treatments

Wedding Bubbles

Rice is out, and birdseed was just too messy—the newest way to wish newlyweds well is with bubbles! I attended a wedding where each guest was given a small bottle of bubbles to blow as the bride and groom left the church. This really isn't a beauty recipe, but it was so much fun I had to include it. I also make up bottles of these bubbles for my daughters to enjoy in the bath and to give as gifts to their friends.

½ cup dish detergent
5 cups cold water
2 tablespoons glycerin
Pipe cleaners

Pour the detergent, water, and glycerin into a clean container and shake or stir gently to mix.

Pipe cleaners make good bubble wands and come in a variety of colors. They are also very inexpensive and can be bent into many different shapes. Make small loops or hearts to blow.

Yield: 40 ounces

BRIDESMAID PARTY

I once gave a bridal shower for the fiancée of one of my husband's friends. I did not know many of the guests well, so I decided to have a manicure party. From experience I have found beauty parties to be great fun and a good way for a group of people to get to know one another. Everyone will appreciate a good manicure, especially before a big social event like a wedding.

The party was a big hit. We discussed everything—including the groom—and never stopped laughing. We went home with beautiful hands and a few new friends, all of us relaxed and looking forward to the big event!

Invitations:

Trace your hand on a piece of heavy construction paper and cut out. Print the party details on these paper hands. You may decorate them as you wish with glitter or stickers, and include an inexpensive cardboard emery board inside each envelope.

(continued)

Party:

Set your table and you'll set the party mood. You may want to use a large towel as a tablecloth or make a painted cloth with handprints. Set at each guest's place a small bowl for soaking nails and a hand towel rather than a napkin. On the table have bowls of cotton balls, swabs, jars of hand cream, and a roll of plastic wrap. You can place a new nail brush marked with each guest's name at each place or ask your friends to bring their own polish and nail care supplies. Serve pickup foods that are easy to eat and drinks that do not have to be opened.

Activities:

Follow the steps on page 128 for The Ultimate Manicure. You may also want to try palm reading—get a good book from the library and study each other's life line. Each guest can take turns reading the palm of the bride-to-be and writing down predictions for her wedding album.

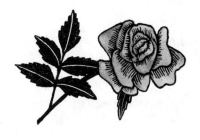

Noble
Nail Polish

1 tablespoon castor oil
1 teaspoon wheat germ oil
1 teaspoon honey
1½ teaspoons sea salt

In ancient times, well-manicured nails were a symbol of culture and civilization. They were a means of distinguishing the laboring commoner from idle aristocrats. This simple mixture of oil, honey, and sea salt, based on an old Egyptian recipe, can be used to give your nails a healthy glow and improve their overall appearance.

Mix the ingredients together and spoon into a clean container. To use: Massage a small amount into your nails and cuticles. Wipe off any excess with a clean soft cloth and lightly buff.

Yield: 2 ounces

Nail-
Strengthening
Oil

1 teaspoon olive oil
1 teaspoon castor oil
¼ teaspoon fresh lemon juice

*C*astor oil and olive oil are both useful in treating dry, brittle nails. They help moisturize the nail and restore its flexibility and strength. This oil can be used for both fingernails and toenails.

Combine all ingredients and mix thoroughly. Pour into a clean bottle with a lid. Remember to shake before using. To use: Rub a small amount of the oil mixture into your nails. Leave on for 5 minutes and wipe off any excess oil. Repeat as often as you like.

Yield: ¾ ounce

The same mask recipes used for the face can be adapted for use on the hands. The consistency for the hand treatment should be a bit thicker because the skin tends to be rougher. Just cut back on the amount of water or other liquid used in the particular recipe. I like to use this mask on my hands in the evening before going to bed. Often, I'll cover my hands with thick cotton gloves to prevent staining and leave the mask on overnight.

Blend the ingredients together into a creamy lotion. Massage the mixture into your hands and cover them with cotton gloves before going to bed. In the morning, remove the gloves, wash your hands with a mild soap, and massage in some hand cream. Store any leftover mask in the refrigerator.

Yield: 2 ounces, enough for 1 treatment

Overnight Hand Mask

½ teaspoon wheat germ oil
1 teaspoon castor oil
½ teaspoon vitamin E oil
2 tablespoons plain yogurt

This rich cream is perfect for massaging into the cuticle at the base of each nail to condition and increase circulation. Massaging this cream daily into your cuticles will keep them soft and help promote healthy nail growth. Keep a small jar next to the telephone, television, or bedside table. Remember to push back your cuticles gently—never cut them.

Combine the ingredients in an ovenproof glass container and heat gently in a double boiler or in the microwave. When all the ingredients have melted, pour the mixture into a clean container. Cool completely before using. To use: Massage a small amount of the cream into each cuticle.

Yield: 2 ounces

Cuticle Cream

2 tablespoons petroleum jelly
2 tablespoons jojoba oil
1 teaspoon anhydrous lanolin or lanolin cream
½ teaspoon grated cocoa butter

The Ultimate Manicure

Your hands are often forgotten when it comes to weekly beauty routines. Many people consider manicures an indulgence or vanity treatment for fancy nails. This just isn't so: Proper hand care is important for everyone, especially very busy people. I like to set aside Sunday evenings for my hands, but anytime that's relaxing can work for you. A good manicure can take up to an hour, but it's time well spent because the results will last all week. Men's hands need care, too! Many couples enjoy sharing this hand treatment.

Steps to follow for beautiful hands:

1. Remove all traces of nail polish.

2. Soak your hands in warm water with a gentle cleanser for ten minutes. I like to use the Honey Cleanser described on page 147, which helps soften your cuticles. Use a gentle nail brush and clean under each nail.

3. Massage a rich hand cream into your hands and cuticles. Gently push back your cuticles with a cotton-tipped orange stick. Never cut your cuticles!

4. File your nails into square ovals, making sure all are the same length.

(continued)

5. Make a hand mask, using your favorite facial mask recipe. I prefer to use sour cream with a bit of honey. Leave the mask on your hands for fifteen to twenty minutes.

6. Rinse off all the mask with warm water followed by cool water.

7. Massage a rich hand cream into your hands. Work from the base of your palm to your fingertips, one finger at a time. Wrap your hands in plastic wrap and let rest for fifteen to twenty minutes or put on cotton gloves before going to bed.

I prefer the "natural" look as opposed to bold colors on my nails. For a bit of color and shine I simply buff with a soft chamois buffer and a bit of cornstarch on each nail. For a hint of color, try a nail "tint" rather than a polish. Mix a bit of red henna with water and brush the solution onto clean, dry nails.

Flower Power Cologne

This is a light, fresh toilet water that combines two of my favorite garden scents—rose and lavender—with fresh herbs and citrus peel for an irresistible scent, perfect for splashing on throughout the day.

2 tablespoons fresh rose petals
2 tablespoons fresh lavender flowers
Peel of 1 lemon (zest only)
1 tablespoon fresh rosemary
1 tablespoon fresh peppermint
2 cups water
1¼ cups vodka

Place the flowers, peel, and herbs in a small saucepan and cover with the water. Simmer on low heat for 5 minutes but do not boil. Cool completely and add the vodka. Pour the mixture into a clean container with a tight-fitting lid and place in a cool, dry location for 2 weeks. Strain off all solids and bottle your cologne in a pretty bottle.

Yield: 16 ounces

Eye Rest Pillow

These pretty silk pillows are a simple and effective way to ease the strain on your eyes. See the pattern on page 249. Once you place the pillow over your eyes, you'll find that the soothing darkness and scent of lavender will refresh and relax you. This is a perfect gift item for thinkers, visionaries, readers, and computer users! I use flaxseeds to fill the pillows because of their long shelf life. They also give a very soft, "fluid" feel to the pillow. Flaxseeds are what linseed oil is made from; they can be found at many health food stores. If you cannot find flaxseeds, however, you may substitute small-grain rice.

2 pieces of 100 percent silk material
5 inches by 9 inches in size (look for silk scarves and lingerie on sale at thrift stores)
1 cup flaxseeds
1 tablespoon dried lavender flowers

With right sides together, sew the two pieces of silk using a ⅝-inch seam allowance and leaving a 1-inch opening on one side. Turn the pillow right side out.

Mix together the flaxseeds and lavender flowers. Using a small funnel, fill the pillow with the seeds and flowers. Stitch the opening closed by hand.

To use: Lie down, place the pillow over your eyes for at least 10 minutes, and relax.

Yield: 1 pillow

Three Musketeers Aftershaves

I have chosen three different aftershaves for Alexandre Dumas's popular musketeers, Athos, Porthos, and Aramis, whose famous line—"One for all and all for one!"—earned them an eternal place in literary history and who are representative of three very distinct types of men.

Athos

Athos was a deep thinker and visionary who commanded great respect from his contemporaries. A born leader, Athos helped ground the group and keep them focused on the task or adventure at hand. For this man, a classic aftershave made with dark rum and fragrant spices.

½ cup vodka
2 tablespoons rum
2 dried bay leaves
¼ teaspoon whole allspice
1 small cinnamon stick
Zest from 1 small orange

Mix all the ingredients together. Pour into a clean jar with a tight-fitting lid. Place the jar in a dark, cool place for 2 weeks. Strain off the liquid and pour into a clean container.

To use: Lightly splash on the face after shaving.

Yield: 4 ounces

Porthos

2 tablespoons witch hazel
2 tablespoons vodka
1/8 teaspoon menthol crystals
Pinch of alum
1/4 teaspoon boric acid powder
1 teaspoon glycerin
1/4 cup water

Porthos had a zest for life. He was fun-loving and the center of any social gathering. Of the three musketeers, Porthos had the best sense of humor. For him an exhilarating menthol after-shave. Both menthol crystals and alum powder are found at most drug stores and many grocery stores in the health care section.

Mix together all the ingredients and pour into a clean bottle with a tight-fitting lid. To use: Lightly splash on the face after shaving.

Yield: 4 ounces

Aramis

1/2 cup vodka
1/2 cup witch hazel
1 tablespoon dried lavender flowers
1 tablespoon dried sage leaves
1 dried bay leaf
4 black peppercorns
1 tablespoon glycerin

Aramis was handsome, religious, and poetic. He was the romantic of the trio, and his charm and passion for life infected all who surrounded him. For him a classic scent with a hint of floral notes.

Mix together all the ingredients. Pour into a clean jar with a tight-fitting lid. Place the jar in a dark, cool place for 2 weeks. Strain off the liquid and discard any solids, then pour into a clean container. To use: Lightly splash on the face after shaving.

Yield: 8 ounces

FATHER'S DAY GIFT

Create a gift box for your father on his special day filled with skin care products you have made. Aftershave is a popular gift for fathers on this day. This year why not make your own for Dad?

Suggested items to include:

Three Musketeers Aftershave (page 131)

New razor

Olive Oil Shaving Cream (page 79)

Lincoln Footbath (page 76)

Colorful washcloth

Wrap each item in newsprint. Paint an old cigar box or shoe box in a wood grain pattern, then write a brief note or poem about your father and glue it to the inside lid of the box. Tie up the whole package with some braided raffia or jute twine and add a few dried bay leaves to the top of the package. I use an office hole punch to put holes in the leaves. You can also sign each child's name on a different leaf.

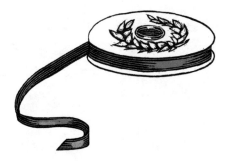

Breath Freshener

1 tablespoon liquid chlorophyll
¼ teaspoon honey

Brushing your teeth decreases mouth odors by 25 percent; brushing your teeth and tongue together decreases odors by 85 percent. Always try to brush after each meal to reduce bad breath and to keep your teeth and gums clean and healthy. Often, however, you may not have the time or the access to a toothbrush. Liquid chlorophyll is a powerful natural deodorant that can sometimes be found in mint flavor. Mixed with a small amount of honey, it makes for a super breath freshener. Just place a drop or two on your tongue when needed.

Mix together the chlorophyll and honey and pour into a small bottle with a dropper or spray top.

Yield: ½ ounce

TRAVEL BEAUTY

The most common symptoms of travel fatigue are exhaustion, dehydration, swelling of the joints, dry skin, sore eyes, and disturbed sleep. When traveling, remember that it is essential to drink plenty of hydrating liquids such as fruit juices, herbal teas, and, of course, water. Drinking lots of liquids has an added benefit: You'll have to leave your seat more often, which in turn helps your circulation. You should take a brief walk or at least stand up and stretch every hour of your trip. Massaging your legs, knees, and ankles will also help your circulation and keep your feet from swelling.

(continued)

Bring along a spritz bottle filled with some scented water (I like rosewater) to keep your hair and skin hydrated and to freshen the air around you. Airplane air can become especially stale and dry on long flights. When flying, you can never have too much moisture! If you wear contact lenses, you may want to give your eyes a rest and opt to use your glasses. Don't forget to slip your toothbrush inside your purse and use it to keep your mouth fresh and clean. After traveling you will want a refreshing bath or shower. Use scented oils and soaps to help relax and refresh you.

Thinking ahead and packing a few simple beauty essentials inside your purse or briefcase will make all the difference in the world, and you will arrive at your destination looking and feeling terrific!

Aromatherapy for Jet Lag

When you travel through different time zones, your internal body clock can become out of synch, causing jet lag. It's been proven that using a combination of natural essential oils in the bath or shower twice a day will assist you in adapting to a new time zone. Essential oils come in very small bottles that can be carried in your purse or briefcase. The appropriate fragrance should be used before starting the day and before going to bed for as many days as the time zones you have passed through. For example, flying from New York to Los Angeles you travel through three different time zones, so you'll use the scented oils for three days to help your body adjust to your new location.

For daytime (to wake up)

2 drops essential oil of
    peppermint
2 drops essential oil of
    eucalyptus

For evening (to go to sleep)

2 drops essential oil of lavender
2 drops essential oil of geranium

When you arrive at your new location, try to stay awake and adjust to the local time. Use the evening oil combination before going to bed.

In the shower: Massage the oil into your torso and around the sinuses before getting into a warm shower. Stay in the shower for 5 minutes. You may mix the oils with some shower gel or light oil if you wish.

In the bath: Pour the scented oils into a warm bath and bathe in the fragrant water for 10 minutes.

Note: If you are anxious when flying, you may want to put a few drops of the evening combination (lavender/geranium) onto a cotton handkerchief and sniff the cloth during the flight to calm your nerves. Sipping chamomile tea will also help; you'll have to pack your own tea bags.

Hotel Room Beauty

Believe it or not, hotel room stays are the perfect time for beauty treatments! There are fewer distractions than in your own home and plenty of clean fluffy towels. I have several friends who travel quite a bit on business and look forward to their hotel "beauty nights." It is the one place they can sleep with conditioner in their hair or read in the bathtub in complete silence. If you're creative, you can find many key beauty ingredients in the average hotel room or have them delivered via room service. Here are a few of my favorites:

Sugar packets: Sugar can make excellent face and body scrubs. Simply sprinkle a bit of sugar into your hand and mix together with water, cleanser, or soap. Scrub lightly to remove any dead skin and surface impurities, and rinse well. Table salt will also work as a body scrub, but don't use it on your face.

Tea bags: Tea bags are wonderful for resting tired, puffy eyes. The caffeine helps reduce swelling. Simply wet the bags with cool water, lie down, and place a bag over your eyelids. Then rest for ten to fifteen minutes. Herbal tea bags make wonderful skin fresheners and fragrant relaxing baths. Tie a few bags under the water faucet of the tub when filling it with warm water. I like using chamomile tea to relax and peppermint tea to wake up.

Mini bar: Beer is great as a setting lotion and final rinse for the hair. White wine and gin can both help ease a bad sunburn, and each makes a nice skin-softening bath. Apply with a clean cloth or cotton pad to your skin or pour a cup or two directly into your bathtub under the running water. Gin and vodka also act as mild skin astringents. Remember to moisturize well after using alcohol-based products because they can dry out your skin. If you have dry or sensitive skin, dilute the alcohol with equal parts of water.

Fruit basket: If you are lucky enough to have a fruit basket delivered to your room, you have the makings for several skin-conditioning facial masks. Bananas, pears, apples, grapes, and strawberries are all wonderful facial mask ingredients. Simply rub a bit of the fruit over your skin or apply a thicker layer of mashed fruit and leave it on for ten to fifteen minutes. Rinse well with tepid water and pat your skin dry.

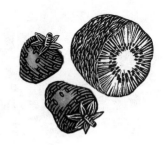

Room service: Save those condiment jars after a room service meal. Mayonnaise and honey both make excellent moisturizing hair treatments. Massage the mayonnaise or honey into your hair and scalp, and cover with a plastic shower cap or plastic laundry bag. Let the conditioner sit for fifteen to twenty minutes before shampooing.

Shampoo, shower gel, conditioner: Pack along a small bottle or two of your favorite scented oil or essential oil and add a few drops to the complimentary toiletries for a bit of aromatherapy. I like to add a bit of lavender oil to the shower gel and pour it in my bath—it's perfect for relaxing after a long day.

Exercise: Besides taking advantage of the hotel gym, use the stairs, participate in exercises shown on television, do yoga in your room, and walk everywhere. Physical activity is relaxing and will help you sleep better. You will also feel healthier after all those restaurant meals you tend to eat while on the road.

BON VOYAGE BASKET

Fill a plastic bag or travel case with a few beauty essentials for yourself or a special friend who is about to take a trip. Whether the person is traveling across the country or around the world, a few new beauty items will make the journey a more enjoyable experience.

Suggested items to include:

Set of essential oils for jet lag (page 135)

Maps of destination

Matterhorn Lip Balm (page 56)

Zanzibar Foot Oil (page 74)

Inflatable neck pillow for napping

Green Tea Skin Toner (page 107)

Wrap each item in tissue paper and place inside a large resealable plastic bag. Tie up the bag with a pretty ribbon and use a travel post-card as a gift label.

Summer Skin and Hair Care

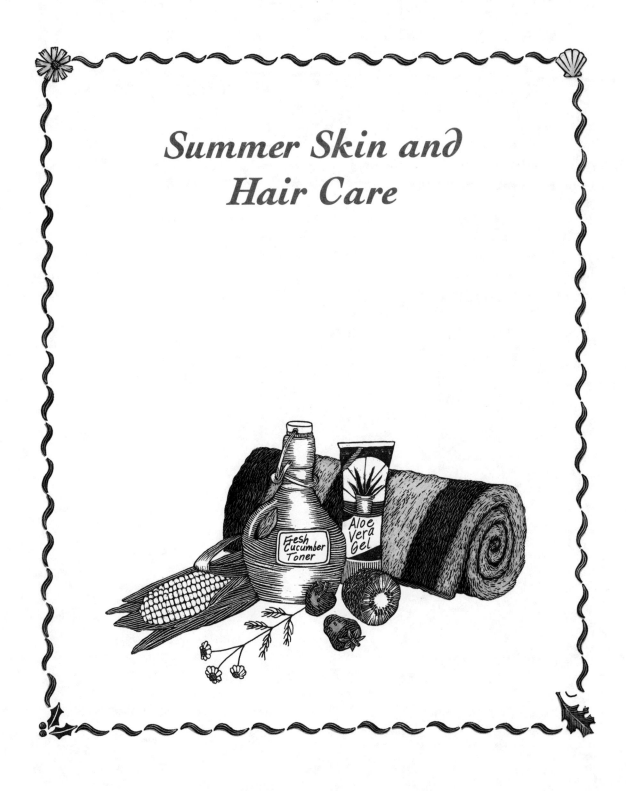

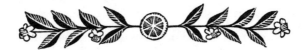

*S*ummer is my favorite season for creating beauty products because fresh ingredients are in abundant supply. This is the time of year to stock up for the other seasons by preserving summer's bounty of herbs, produce, and flowers. My kitchen and garage are decorated with drying bundles of flowers and herbs. Each windowsill has a dish of rose petals or citrus peels drying in the sun for later use. (You can find instructions for drying your own herbs and flowers on page 33.) Grower's markets and roadside farm stands are some of the best sources for fresh produce and flowers during the summer. My daughters and I love to visit local farms in our area where we can pick our own fresh fruits and berries—raspberries and peaches are our favorite. And we make at least a weekly visit to our local organic produce grocers, which always inspires a new beauty treatment or two.

Summer sun protection is crucial. Always protect your skin and hair from overexposure to the sun when you venture outside for more than twenty minutes at a time. The safest time to go out in the sun is when your shadow is taller than you, in the morning before 10:00 and in the afternoon after 3:00, because the sun is not directly overhead and at its strongest. The sun emits harmful ultraviolet rays of two types. UV A rays penetrate the dermis (the second layer of skin) and contribute to skin damage and premature aging; UV B are the burning rays that turn skin red and give you a sunburn. Use a good sunscreen every day for protection and apply it to your skin generously fifteen to twenty minutes before going out. Medications such as antibiotics, antihistamines, and birth control pills may increase your sensitivity to the sun, so check with your physician or pharmacist to see what level of protection you will need.

Warmer weather also speeds up your metabolism, which translates into more active oil glands and, hence, oilier skin. You may need to clean your skin more often, so carry along a mild astringent or toner in your purse or summer tote. Use facial masks more frequently, perhaps twice a week. A good mask will help deep-clean your skin and allow it to "breathe." One of my favorite summer masks is cold sour cream. Cleansing scrubs are a good way to keep summer skin glowing; just remember that they can make your skin more sensitive to the sun.

Summer weather, salt water, and chlorine are especially drying to your hair. Deep-conditioning treatments should be used weekly to restore moisture to your hair and scalp. My favorite summer treatment is the simple Banana Hair Conditioner described on page 172. Hair can also get sunburned, which causes it to lose its shine and break easily. Wearing scarves and hats will protect your hair from the sun and wind. (They'll also help protect your face from UV damage.) Find a pretty, plain straw hat and make it your signature this summer by decorating it with ribbon, flowers, seashells, or raffia in your favorite colors.

Your feet also need more attention this season because they are constantly exposed—going barefoot is what summer is all about! Weekly pedicures will keep your feet looking and feeling their best. See the instructions for The Ultimate Pedicure on page 188.

Outsmart the heat and humidity of those dog days of summer by dressing in loose, natural-fiber clothing. Shower after you exercise and use powder to absorb perspiration. My recipe for Cooling Cinnamon Body Powder on page 179 is a good one to try. Make a body powder that includes rice flour because ground rice contains the UV-ray filtering agent gamma oryzanol.

Summer beauty products also make welcome gifts. Make up a special Summer Tote Bag like the one on page 151 or the Country Beauty Basket on page 155 to give as a hostess gift or thank-you for a special friend. I like to put together birthday baskets that include several bath products, a scented candle, a fruit iced tea (such as mango-hibiscus) and a relaxation tape or CD.

For a description of common summer ingredients and where to find them, see page 20.

Summer Scrubs

*S*un exposure thickens the outer layer of the skin. This can block oil glands and cause breakouts to occur. One way to keep your skin healthy and glowing is to use a face and body scrub once or twice a week. If you have sensitive skin, use a very gentle scrub such as wheat germ. I have seen recipes and products that call for ground pumice. Please do not use these, especially on your face—the pumice is just too harsh. Oily skin types should mix the scrubs with a little water or soap. Those with dry skin should use cleansing cream or oil. Sour cream and yogurt work well for all skin types. For gift-giving, layer a clear jar with one or two of these scrubs—blue and yellow cornmeal look nice together.

FOR THE FACE AND BODY:

Finely ground citrus peels
Finely ground apricot, peach, or nectarine kernels
   (inside pit)
Cornmeal
Oatmeal
Wheat germ—especially good for sensitive skin

FOR THE BODY ONLY:

Ground avocado stone (pit)
Ground almonds
Coarse salt
Ground sunflower seeds (shelled)

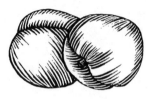

Cucumber and Chamomile Cleanser

This is a mild nonsoap cleanser that is perfect for delicate or sensitive skin. Cucumber juice, chamomile flowers, and aloe vera gel are all gentle astringents and soothing to the skin. Because of the mildness of this cleanser it can be used more than once a day. If you do not have fresh flowers in your garden, you may substitute tea bags made from 100 percent chamomile flowers.

2 tablespoons fresh cucumber juice (see Note)

2 tablespoons fresh chamomile flower heads or 1 tablespoon dried

1 cup distilled water

1 tablespoon glycerin

1 tablespoon aloe vera gel

Make a strong infusion of the chamomile flowers and water, and let cool. When cool, strain off all solids. Mix together the cucumber juice, chamomile tea, glycerin, and aloe vera gel.

To use: Saturate a clean cotton pad with the cleanser and run over your skin. Repeat if necessary. You may rinse with cool water and use a light moisturizer. Store in the refrigerator because cucumber juice spoils easily.

Note: To make fresh cucumber juice puree a fresh cucumber in a blender or food processor and strain the green juice.

Yield: 9 ounces

Victorian Cleansing Powder

This is one of my favorite nonsoap cleansers. It has a lovely scent and turns a wonderful shade of lavender when wet. Extremely gentle and perfect for cleaning all skin types, this cleansing powder is an elegant gift fit for a lady. Pour this powder into a pretty jar and tie a lace handkerchief over the lid with a satin ribbon. You can also tie an antique silver spoon to the jar for scooping out the powder.

2 tablespoons oats
1 teaspoon dried lavender flowers
1 teaspoon dried red rose petals
2 tablespoons white kaolin clay
   (sometimes called China clay,
   found at natural food stores and
   some pharmacies)

In a coffee or spice grinder, finely grind the oats, lavender, and rose petals. The mixture should resemble bread flour in consistency. Depending on the size of your grinder, you may have to grind the mixture in small portions. Stir the white clay into the ground mixture and pour the cleansing powder into a clean airtight container.

To use: Combine about 1 teaspoon of the powder with some water in your hand to form a smooth paste. Gently clean your skin with this paste and rinse well with cool water.

Yield: 3 ounces

Honey Cleanser

Honey gently softens and cleanses the skin. This is a mild nonsoap cleanser that works well for dry skin types. It's not at all sticky and can be used as either a facial cleanser or bath gel. I like to fill empty honey squeeze bottles (especially those bears!) with this cleanser. Tie a bow around the neck, and it is a perfect addition to a bath gift basket.

¼ cup honey
1 tablespoon liquid soap
½ cup glycerin

Mix together all ingredients and pour into a clean bottle. Remember to use nonbreakable containers if you are going to be using it in the tub or shower.

Yield: 6 ounces

Sweet Corn Astringent

2 tablespoons fresh corn milk
   (made by grating a fresh ear
   of corn into a bowl and straining
   off the milky white liquid; an
   average ear of corn will yield
   approximately 2 tablespoons
   of fluid)
2 tablespoons distilled water
2 tablespoons vodka
2 tablespoons witch hazel

*T*ender and succulent, fresh sweet corn is a classic summer treat. This mild astringent uses corn "milk" to cleanse and refresh the skin. Fresh corn contains fat, which makes the astringent milder and not as dehydrating for those with dry skin, like me. If you have extremely dry skin, substitute more water for the vodka. I use this product after washing my face to keep it soft and smooth.

Stir together all the ingredients and pour into a clean container with a lid.
   To use: Apply to the skin with a clean cotton ball.

Yield: 4 ounces

New Zealand Kiwi Astringent

1 cup boiling water
1 ripe kiwi fruit, peeled and mashed
1 tablespoon vodka

*"K*iwi" is slang for someone from New Zealand. It's also the commercial name for Chinese gooseberries. These small brown fruits are now grown throughout the United States and are easily found at better grocery stores year-round. New Zealanders know that the kiwi fruit, like other sweet citrus fruits, is a natural astringent. After washing your face, simply squeeze the juice from a kiwi onto a cotton ball and apply as a cooling and refreshing skin toner. Then rinse thoroughly. (This is especially therapeutic for oily skin.) I find straight kiwi juice a little too acidic for my skin, so I use this recipe, which is milder because it contains more water.

Pour the boiling water over the mashed kiwi fruit in a heavy ceramic bowl and let sit until cool (about 20–30 minutes).

Strain the mixture well to remove all fruit solids and seeds. I usually strain twice, once with a fine metal strainer and then with a paper coffee filter. Add the vodka to the liquid and stir.

To use: Apply to the skin with a clean cotton pad. You may rinse your face with cool water if you have sensitive skin.

Yield: 8 ounces

Fruit-Tea Freshener

Walk down the tea aisle of your local grocery store, and you will be amazed at the number of teas available today, especially caffeine-free fruit teas. These come in a wide range of flavors, such as cranberry, raspberry, mango, peach, and kiwi-strawberry. The fruit teas make wonderful skin fresheners. For a quick pick-me-up on hot summer days, store the freshener in the refrigerator.

1 cup boiling water
2 fruit tea bags of your choice
  (I like to use kiwi-strawberry)
1 tablespoon witch hazel (optional)

Pour the boiling water over the tea bags in a ceramic heat-resistant bowl. Allow the tea bags to steep for several hours, or until the mixture has cooled completely.

Add witch hazel to the infusion. You may want to strain the solution if you see bits of tea at the bottom of the container. I do this by pouring the liquid through a paper coffee filter.

Bottle the fruit-tea freshener and enjoy. Use a clean cotton ball to apply or use a spray bottle to splash on your skin.

Yield: 8 ounces

Fresh Cucumber Toner

¼ cup fresh cucumber juice
    (see Note)
2 tablespoons witch hazel
2 tablespoons distilled water
1 tablespoon vodka

*C*ucumber juice is a natural astringent that also makes a mild tonic for sunburned skin. Fresh cucumber juice is extremely delicate and spoils easily, and adding witch hazel and vodka helps extend its shelf life. Store the finished product in the refrigerator to make it last for a few weeks. This recipe is good for all skin types.

Mix together all the ingredients and pour into a clean bottle with a lid.

To use: Apply to your skin with a clean cotton ball. (It can also be sprayed on the skin.)

Note: To make fresh cucumber juice puree a fresh cucumber in a blender or food processor and strain the green juice.

Yield: 4 ounces

Royal Rose Toner

1 tablespoon dried rose petals
    (or any fragrant dried rose
    petals)
1 cup white wine vinegar
½ cup rosewater

*T*he exquisite rose is without a doubt the queen of the flower kingdom. Since antiquity the rose has been the symbol of romance and beauty. Because roses are naturally astringent and remove oil and dirt from the skin, they are a key ingredient in many beauty products. This mildly acidic toner will remove all traces of soap and cleanser from your skin after washing.

Mix together the rose petals and vinegar and let sit for 2 weeks. Strain well and stir in the rosewater. Pour into a pretty bottle. Spray on or apply to your skin with a clean cotton ball.

Yield: 12 ounces

SUMMER TOTE BAG

A great gift idea for a visiting friend or relative this summer is a new tote bag, filled with beauty essentials, for taking along to the beach or pool.

Suggested items to include:

Hair Conditioning Clay (page 167)
Island Lip Gloss (page 160)
Hat or cotton scarf
Minty Astringent (page 152)
Wooden comb for wet hair
Sunshine Cream (page 182)

Sew or purchase a canvas tote bag that you can personalize and decorate with fabric paints and markers. Wrap each gift in brightly colored paper or cellophane and place inside the bag. Using cotton cord or jute, tie a bunch of silk or fresh flowers to the tote bag's handles to keep them together.

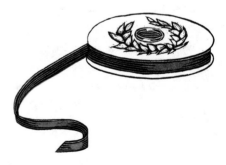

Minty Astringent

3 tablespoons fresh mint leaves of
    your choice or 1½ tablespoons
    dried
1 cup witch hazel

*M*int has always been one of my favorite herbs. I love growing this herb because it is practically foolproof—it seems to flourish when ignored. Mint comes in a variety of scents, which makes for an endless supply of minty astringents and other beauty products. In my own garden I have such varieties as eau de cologne, pineapple, chocolate, peppermint, lavender, orange, and spearmint, all of which work well in this recipe.

Mix together the mint leaves and witch hazel and let sit for 1 week in a dark, dry place. After 1 week, strain off all solids and bottle in a clean container. To use: Apply to the skin using a clean cotton ball or spray with a small spray bottle.

Yield: 8 ounces

Herb Garden Astringent

1 cup water
½ cup vodka
¼ cup of your favorite herbs, such
    as sage, yarrow, chamomile,
    rosemary, lemon balm,
    peppermint, spearmint, basil,
    and lavender
¼ cup witch hazel

*T*his recipe gives you a chance to utilize your garden and your own creativity. Go outside early in the morning just after the morning dew has dried and gather up bunches of your favorite herbs and flowers. You will want to make several batches, trying different combinations of herbs. Keep notes if you want to recreate your favorite combinations or make an extra batch for gift-giving. Label your bottles with a photo from your garden, using a color copier to reproduce your favorite photo image. Attach your custom label to the bottle using a glue stick or tie on with a scrap of cotton cord.

Mix together all the ingredients. Place in a jar with a tight-fitting lid and let sit for 2 weeks. Strain and pour into a clean bottle.

Yield: 16 ounces

Watermelon Toner

Watermelon contains a high amount of vitamins A, B, and C, all of which keep skin healthy and glowing. This aromatic toner is rose-colored and looks lovely in a clear corked bottle. For gift-giving, you may want to make a watermelon-shaped label or use some red paper ribbon with black seeds drawn on the ends.

2 tablespoons fresh watermelon juice (see Note)
1 tablespoon vodka
2 tablespoons witch hazel
2 tablespoons distilled water

Combine the watermelon juice with the remaining ingredients and stir well. Pour into a clean container. To use: Apply to skin with a clean cotton pad.

Note: Make fresh watermelon juice by processing watermelon in a blender or food processor and straining to remove all solids.

Yield: 4 ounces

Helianthus Body Lotion

Helianthus *is the Latin word for sunflower. Sunflower seed oil is a popular cooking oil and is easily found at your local grocery store. This pale yellow oil contains vitamin E and makes a splendid all-over body lotion. Pour the finished lotion into a bottle, wrap the top with some jute cord, and attach a silk or dried sunflower.*

⅛ teaspoon borax powder
½ cup distilled water
½ cup sunflower oil
½ tablespoon grated beeswax

Combine the borax powder and water and stir well. Set aside.

Mix together the oil and beeswax in a heat-resistant container. Heat gently in a water bath or microwave 1–2 minutes, until the wax is melted.

Heat the water solution until it is roughly the same temperature as the oil mixture.

Pour the hot water and borax into a blender and start mixing on low speed. Add the oil and beeswax mixture in a slow, steady, thin stream. When all the oil mixture has been added, turn the blender on high for 2 minutes. (This can also be done by hand. Add the oil to the water and whip with a wire whisk for 2 minutes.)

Let the lotion cool completely. You should have a light white lotion. Pour into a clean container and label.

Yield: 8 ounces

Peach Cold Cream

¼ teaspoon borax powder
1 tablespoon water
¼ cup peach kernel oil (you may also use apricot kernel oil or almond oil)
1 tablespoon grated beeswax
1 tablespoon fresh peach juice made by straining the pulp of a fresh peach
1–2 drops peach fragrance (optional)

Peaches have long been a symbol of beauty, and this simple, fragrant cream will keep your skin glowing and beautiful. Fresh peach juice is a natural emollient and a wonderful salve. You can make a simple scrub from this ointment by adding some crushed peach kernels (the almond-shaped nut inside the peach pit). I like to spread this cream all over my face before showering and let it soak in for twenty minutes. It is guaranteed to give you a peaches-and-cream complexion!

Dissolve the borax powder in the water and set aside.

Place the peach kernel oil and beeswax in a heat-resistant container and heat gently in a water bath or the microwave until the beeswax is melted.

When the beeswax is melted, gently heat the water and borax solution either in the same water bath or in a microwave oven.

Add the peach juice to the water solution and slowly pour into the beeswax-oil mixture in a thin, steady stream, stirring constantly. You can also pour the mixture in a blender and mix on high until well blended.

Pour the thick cream into a container and allow to cool completely. Stir a few drops of peach fragrance into the mixture if you desire a stronger scent. The cold cream will thicken as it cools. To speed up this process you can refrigerate the finished cream.

Yield: 3 ounces

COUNTRY BEAUTY BASKET

Create a country beauty basket by lining a picnic basket with bandanna scarves or gingham fabric. Fill the basket with farm-fresh country beauty products such as Peach Cold Cream (page 154) Watermelon Toner (page 153), yellow cornmeal to be used as a face and body scrub, oatmeal that can be added to the bath, and fresh flowers and herbs. This basket makes a perfect gift for a city friend who dreams of living in the country.

Fine Line Lotion

Vitamin E oil is a time-honored treatment for fine lines and wrinkles. Some women feel that alone it is a little too heavy and sticky, especially for daytime wear, so I've created a recipe that combines the richness of vitamin E oil with rosewater for a lighter texture.

¼ teaspoon vitamin E oil
1 teaspoon almond oil
1 teaspoon rosewater

Mix all ingredients together. Pour into a small, clean bottle. You may have to shake the bottle before applying to remix the lotion because the oil and water will separate.

Yield: ½ ounce

Queen Bee Cold Cream

½ tablespoon bee pollen
1 tablespoon distilled water
¼ cup glycerin
¼ cup grated beeswax
½ cup light oil (almond or
    sunflower work well)

This is a splendid cold cream containing beeswax and bee pollen, both of which soften and moisturize. I like to use it in the evening to remove makeup and cleanse my skin. Local beekeepers are a good source of beeswax and pollen, but you may also purchase bee pollen at many health food stores. Bee pollen is believed to promote healing and help treat skin blemishes. This cream has a warm yellow color and a mild honey scent.

Mix together the bee pollen and water, and stir to dissolve the pollen. Set aside.

Mix together the glycerin, beeswax, and oil, and heat until the wax is melted.

Pour the oil mixture in a blender and slowly add the pollen and water mixture. Blend on high for 1 minute. Pour into a clean container and allow to cool completely.

Yield: 6 ounces

Summer Cleansing Mask

¼ cup sour cream
2 tablespoons oatmeal

This is a simple facial treatment that deep-cleanses the skin and removes any dead skin cells from the surface. Sour cream is one of my favorite beauty ingredients, and I like to do a sour cream facial weekly to keep my skin really clean and glowing. It is also especially cooling on a hot summer day.

Mix together the sour cream and oatmeal. Massage into your face and neck, and leave on for 20 minutes. Rinse with warm water, then cool water. Refrigerate any leftover masque.

Yield: 2 ounces, enough for 1 or 2 treatments

Farmer's Market Facials

One of my favorite activities during the summer growing season is visiting the various farmer's or grower's markets that seem to pop up along the roadside in many communities. The fresh fruits, vegetables, and flowers are all at their seasonal best, and many are grown organically, which is why I prefer to use them to create my natural beauty products. Here is a list of simple facial masks for you to create using farm-fresh ingredients:

Corn: The high protein and fat content of corn soothes dry skin. Grate an ear of corn and strain off the milky liquid. Pat this on your skin and let sit for 15–20 minutes, then rinse with cool water.

Raspberries: Fresh raspberries make a good after-sun facial mask. Lightly mashed, their juice soothes and refreshes tired skin. You may want to mix the fresh juice with a small amount of honey. Spread the mixture on your skin and let sit for 15–20 minutes, then rinse with warm water.

Melon: Honeydew, cantaloupe, and watermelon all make light toning facial masks. Melons contain vitamins A, B, and C, which keep skin healthy and glowing. Cut paper-thin slices of fresh melon and place on your face and neck (you will have to lie down). Let sit for 15–20 minutes, then rinse with cool water.

Tomato: Tomatoes are mildly acidic, so they make a good astringent mask for oily skin. They are also a good cure for blackheads. Using a clean cotton ball or pastry brush, spread a thin, even layer of fresh tomato juice over your face and neck. Let sit for 10 minutes, then rinse well with tepid water. For sensitive skin you may want to use yellow tomatoes since they contain less acid than the red varieties.

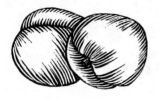

Peaches: Peaches are especially soothing for dry skin. Mash a fresh peach and combine with a bit of fresh cream or yogurt to make a smooth paste. Using a clean cotton ball or pastry brush, spread the mixture over your face and let sit for 15–20 minutes. Rinse well with tepid water.

Fresh Strawberry Mask

½ cup fresh strawberries
1 tablespoon fresh milk
1 tablespoon rice flour or
    cornstarch

Beginning in the early summer and into the fall, strawberries make their appearance in the market. What you may not know is that they make an excellent skin-softening facial mask. A member of the rose family, strawberries contain salicylic acid, which rids the skin of dead cells, allowing it to absorb moisture more efficiently. Strawberries also have a mild bleaching effect on the skin and help heal blemishes.

Mix together all the ingredients to make a smooth paste. Spread over your face and neck and let sit for 20 minutes. Rinse with warm water and pat your skin dry. Refrigerate any leftover mask and discard it if the milk sours.

Yield: 4 ounces, enough for 1 or 2 facial masks

Papaya Anti-Wrinkle Facial

Using natural fruit acids and enzymes to remove dead skin cells is a popular facial treatment in many salons. Skin will look and feel younger and smoother when the top layer of dead skin cells has been removed; this is often called a "fruit peel." Papaya contains a natural enzyme called papain. The greener the papaya, the higher the enzyme content. Care should be exercised when using this treatment. If left on the skin too long, it can be extremely drying. Do not leave on your face for more than five minutes and rinse thoroughly.

2 tablespoons mashed papaya
1 teaspoon aloe vera gel

Mix together the papaya and aloe vera gel to make a smooth paste. Apply to your clean face and neck and let sit for 5 minutes. Rinse with cool water and moisturize well.

Yield: 1 ounce, enough for 1 facial treatment

Beeswax Lip Balm

This is a very simple but effective lip balm. Many of my friends tell me that when they use beeswax on their lips, they do not have to reapply it as often as name brand ointments. It is long lasting and keeps lips feeling soft and smooth.

2 tablespoons grated beeswax
½ tablespoon coconut oil

In a double boiler or microwave, gently melt the beeswax and coconut oil together and stir well. Pour into a clean lip balm container or small plastic box and allow to cool completely.

Yield: 1½ ounces

Island
Lip Gloss

1 teaspoon grated cocoa butter
1 teaspoon coconut oil
1 teaspoon macadamia nut oil
1 teaspoon light sesame oil
⅛ teaspoon vitamin E oil

This is a tropical treat for summer lips that contains the finest island beauty ingredients, including cocoa butter, coconut oil, and macadamia nut oil. I recently discovered macadamia nut oil and love it! It's lighter than many other oils and is easily absorbed into skin and lips. It also adds a mild nutty scent and flavor to this lip gloss. If you cannot find macadamia nut oil, substitute light olive or almond oil. The vitamin E oil in this recipe acts as a natural preservative.

Place all ingredients in an ovenproof container and heat the mixture in the microwave or in a hot, but not boiling, water bath until the cocoa butter and coconut oil are melted.

Stir the mixture well and pour into a small clean container. Lip gloss containers or small plastic boxes work well. Allow the mixture to cool completely.

Spread a small amount onto your lips. This gloss can be worn over or under colored lipstick. Store the gloss in a cool, dry place.

Yield: ½ ounce

Star-Spangled Shower Gel

This is an exhilarating and uplifting morning bath and shower gel. Because the large amount of peppermint oil in the recipe can act as a stimulant, I would not recommend it for evening use. Pour this pale pink liquid into a plastic bottle with a stopper. For gift-giving, decorate with stars or package together with red, white, and blue washcloths.

Mix together all ingredients and pour into a clean container with a lid or stopper. To use: Squeeze a small amount on a clean washcloth or sponge and massage into your skin. Rinse well.

Yield: 8 ounces

½ cup liquid soap (clear or white)
1 tablespoon raspberry vinegar
 (purchased or see recipe below)
¼ teaspoon peppermint oil
½ cup distilled water

Raspberry Vinegar

This is a simple fruit vinegar you can use in beauty recipes or by itself in the bath. Other fresh berries, such as blueberries, blackberries, and huckleberries, also work well.

Heat the vinegar to near boiling. Stir in the fresh raspberries. Remove from the heat and let cool. Strain out all solids and pour into a clean container.

Yield: 8 ounces

1 cup white wine vinegar
½ cup fresh raspberries

Aphrodite Ocean Bath

4 cups coarse sea salt (available at natural food stores and many grocery stores)

*A*phrodite, the Greek goddess of love and beauty, was born of sea foam off the coast of Cyprus. Seawater, with its heavy concentration of salts and minerals, has proven regenerative powers. Nicks, cuts, and blemishes heal quickly when bathed in it. Prepare this bath at home and feel like a Greek goddess yourself. For gift-giving, fill a glass jar with sea salt and tie a seashell onto the lid to use as a spoon.

Add ½ cup of salt to a bath that is a little below body temperature, around 97 degrees. Powdered seaweed (available at natural food stores and Asian markets) may be added if desired. Rinse after bathing.

Yield: 32 ounces, enough for 8 baths

Sea Salt Bath

¼ cup sea salt
¼ cup dried dulse
¼ cup Epsom salts
¼ cup baking soda

*W*hen you can't get to the ocean as often as you'd like, take a therapeutic mini-vacation in your own tub. You'll feel the same great results! These salts provide that much needed "escape" to the sea. Dried seaweed added to your bath helps rid the body of toxins and boosts circulation. Asian markets are a good source for finding a variety of dried seaweed. I like to use dried dulse because it has a pretty red color and has a milder scent than other sea plants.

Mix together all the ingredients and pour into a clean dry container. To use: Pour ¼ cup into the tub under running water.

For a great gift: These salts and the Aphrodite Ocean Bath (recipe above) both look nice packaged in a large seashell or pretty jar. Use a hot-glue gun or craft glue to attach seashells to the jar lid. Tie up the package with a small cotton rope or beautiful sea-colored ribbon.

Yield: 8 ounces, enough for 4 baths

Layered Bath Herbs

This is a beautiful gift for the bath and is quite simple to make. Just layer your favorite dried herbs and flower petals in a clear jar; they are also pretty mixed together. The herbs can be cast individually into the tub or placed in a large tea ball or muslin bag and tied under the running water tap for a refreshing bath.

Layer the dried ingredients in a clean jar until the jar is filled and cover with a decorative lid or cork stopper. Tie a large tea ball to the jar with a pretty ribbon or a scrap of raffia. Label your jar with ingredients and instructions to fill the tea ball and let float in the bath or place under the running tap. Make sure to keep a jar for your own bath.

Yield: depends on the amount of herbs used

Choose 3 or 5 items from the following list:
Lavender flowers
Rose petals (a variety of colors look nice)
Rose hips
Hibiscus flowers
Chamomile flowers
Mint
Basil
Rosemary

Lauren's Lavender Bath

1/4 cup fresh lavender flowers or
2 tablespoons dried

My daughter Lauren loves the scent of fresh lavender flowers—she likes to handpick the flowers for this fragrant bath and fills the bath bag herself. Lavender is ideal for the bathtub because it promotes tranquility and relaxation. Scientific evidence shows that certain aromatherapy scents, and lavender in particular, increase alpha waves in the back of the head associated with a more relaxed state. A lavender bath will also soothe sunburn and insect bites. To Lauren, this information is all quite incidental—she just thinks it "smells really nice."

Fill a cotton or muslin bag with fresh lavender flowers and hang the bag under the tub faucet. Run a warm bath, allowing the water to flow through the bath bag. After the bathtub is full, give the bath bag a few good squeezes to release all the fragrant lavender oil into the tub, then lie back and relax.

Yield: 2 ounces, enough for 1 bath

Maui Pineapple Body Scrub

Outer peel of fresh pineapple cut
into strips or wedges

Whenever I serve fresh pineapple, I always save the outer rind to use later as a body scrub in the bath or shower. Pineapple contains an active enzyme called bromelain, which cleanses and rejuvenates dull skin by removing dead skin cells and surface dirt and oils. This fruity scrub leaves your skin with a soft, smooth feel. Remember to moisturize well after bathing because this treatment can be drying to your skin. Because it's slightly acidic, this scrub should not be used on your face.

RELAXATION BASKET

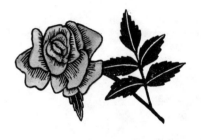

Taking time out and relaxing is something we often forget to do in today's busy world. Relaxing actually boosts our energy level and refreshes both mind and body. Give this basket to someone in your life who could really use a soothing break!

Suggested items to include:

Aphrodite Ocean Bath (page 162)

Bath pillow

Lauren's Lavender Bath (page 164)

Lullaby Oil (page 67)

Relaxation Tape (page 168)

A box of chamomile tea

Fill a basket with beautiful dried flowers and herbs that can be strewn into the bathwater and enjoyed. I like to use rose buds, lavender flowers, and bay leaves. Tie a bit of raffia or linen ribbon around each item and write an inspiring word on each one. Words I like to use: allow, delight, embrace, support, relax, rest, dream, and listen. Nestle the presents inside the fragrant materials, wrap the whole basket in a piece of cellophane or tissue paper, and tie with a ribbon. Tack or glue a few dried herbs onto a large gift tag and write your friend's name or a meaningful message across the tag.

Use the pineapple peels in the shower as you would a sponge or loofah to scrub your body and exfoliate dead skin cells. Wrap any extra peels and refrigerate, or freeze for longer storage.

Yield: 1 to 2 whole body treatments per whole pineapple

Mahalo Massage Oil

½ cup macadamia nut oil (if you cannot find, substitute light sesame oil)

½ teaspoon vitamin E oil

2–3 drops exotic fragrance such as frangipani, sandalwood, or ylang-ylang

*H*awaii abounds in exotic fruits and nuts, and is especially famous for its macadamia nuts. This aromatic island massage oil will have your partner saying "Mahalo," which is Hawaiian for "thank you"! You can also use this natural oil after a shower or bath to give your skin softness and strength.

Pour all the ingredients into a clean bottle and shake well. Store in a dark, dry spot, keep corked between uses, and shake to remix.

Yield: 4 ounces

Summer Massage Spirits

During the summer months, some people prefer to use alcohol for massages because it is light and very cooling on hot days. This is a scented rubbing alcohol that is refreshing and relaxing. Use your favorite herbs to evoke a particular effect (see below). Remember to follow up with a good all-over body lotion, as the alcohol can dry out your skin.

Stimulating Herbs	Relaxing Herbs
Rosemary	Chamomile
Oregano	Lavender
Mint	Basil

2 cups vodka
2 teaspoons glycerin
½ teaspoon castor oil
2 tablespoons dried or ¼ cup fresh herbs (see list at left)

Mix together all the ingredients and allow to sit for 1 week. Strain off the herbs and pour the clear liquid into a clean container with a tight-fitting lid. Use to massage the body in place of massage oil or as an after-bath splash.

Yield: 16 ounces

Hair-Conditioning Clay

This is a rich conditioning hair treatment that can be used before or after shampooing your hair. It acts as a deep cleanser and adds body and bounce to fine or limp hair. Jojoba bean oil has become very popular recently because it is very similar to our bodies' own natural oils. It is easily found in many natural food stores.

¼ cup jojoba oil
1 tablespoon coconut oil
2 tablespoons white clay (kaolin or China clay)
½ cup water

Heat together the jojoba and coconut oils until the coconut oil has melted. This doesn't take long, perhaps 1 to 2 minutes. Combine the melted oils with the clay and water, and stir well, then pour into a clean container and label.

To use: Wet hair and pour a small amount into your palm (approximately 1 tablespoon). Massage thoroughly into your hair and scalp. Wrap your head with plastic and cover with a towel turban-style. Let the conditioner sit on your hair for 10–15 minutes, then shampoo as usual. You may have to shampoo twice to remove the conditioner. If the mixture separates between uses, simply run hot water over the closed container to remelt the coconut oil and shake gently to mix.

Yield: 6 ounces

Summer Braid Gel

This simple natural styling gel will keep your summer braids or any hairdo affected by the humidity in place. Flaxseeds—small, shiny brown seeds that are found in health and nutrition stores—are an important source of linseed oil. When soaked in water, they create a gelatinous solution that gives hair extra body and lift.

2 tablespoons flax seeds
1 cup water

Mix together the flaxseeds and water in a small saucepan and bring to a boil. Remove from the heat and let sit for 15 minutes. Strain the clear jellylike liquid and allow to cool completely. You can add a few drops of your favorite fragrance or essential oil to the cooled mixture if you prefer the recipe scented.

Pour into a clean container with a lid. It will thicken if left uncovered.

To use: Simply apply a small amount as you would any setting or styling gel. I like to use it on wet hair before blow-drying, but it works equally well on dry hair.

Yield: 8 ounces

Conditioning Hair Packs

Sun, wind, chlorine, and salt water are surefire ingredients for dry, damaged hair. To keep your summer tresses healthy and restore moisture to your hair, you should use a deep hair-conditioning pack once a week. This recipe is for normal hair but can be easily adapted for both dry and oily hair types.

½ cup mayonnaise
½ avocado, mashed

Mix together all the ingredients. Rinse hair with warm water and massage mixture into hair and scalp. Cover your hair with plastic wrap—a plastic bag or an old shower cap. Let sit for 15–20 minutes, then, without rinsing, shampoo and style your hair as usual.

Extra-dry or damaged hair: Add 1 tablespoon of coconut oil.

Oily hair: Add 1 to 2 teaspoons of lemon juice.

Yield: 4 ounces, enough for 1 treatment

Philippine Conditioning Hair Rinse

1 fresh coconut
4 cups boiling water

In the tropical Philippine Islands, women use fresh coconut milk to keep their hair soft and shiny. You can purchase coconut milk at the market, but I like to make my own. This is a perfect conditioning rinse for sun-damaged hair because coconut milk is rich in cream and oil. When choosing fresh coconuts, always shake them—you should feel and hear the coconut water swish inside the shell.

Preheat your oven to 400°F. Pierce the eyes (three spots located on one end) of the coconut with an ice pick or sharp skewer. Drain the coconut water and save; an average coconut will yield approximately ½ cup.

Bake the coconut for 15 minutes, then remove it from the oven and place on a solid work surface such as a wooden cutting board. With a hammer, hit the coconut until the shell breaks away and you're left with just the coconut meat.

Rinse the coconut meat and slice into small pieces. There's no need to remove the brown outer peel to make the milk for this treatment. Place these pieces in a blender or food processor, add the reserved coconut water, and chop finely.

Place the coconut meat in a large ceramic bowl and cover with boiling water. Let sit for 30 minutes.

Strain the mixture, and you have coconut milk. You may want to save the solids to use as a body scrub.

Store this rinse in the refrigerator. The coconut cream will float to the top, so stir before using.

To use: Pour approximately 1 cup over freshly shampooed hair as a final rinse. If you have very dry hair, leave in without rinsing. Other hair types may want to rinse with water to remove the excess oil.

Gift idea: Save your empty shells for packaging small gifts. Fill one shell half with tissue paper, tuck a few small items inside, and cover with the other half. Keep the shell halves together with a bit of raffia or fabric ribbon, and you'll have a great gift package.

Yield: 32 ounces, enough for 3 treatments

Swimming Pool Hair Care

Swimming is one of the great joys of summer, but the chlorine and chemicals used in many public swimming pools can be harsh and damaging to hair. When swimming, wear a bathing cap when possible. Wetting your hair with fresh water before you swim will also keep it from soaking up too much chlorine water. Always remember to rinse your hair well after swimming. You may have to bring a bottle of water with you to the pool for just this reason. My friend Diane has beautiful blond hair, and so do both of her daughters. In order to keep their hair from turning green, they use this recipe after a day at the pool.

2 tablespoons baking soda
¼ cup fresh lemon juice
1 teaspoon mild shampoo

Mix together all the ingredients until well blended. Wet hair and massage mixture well into hair and scalp, making sure hair ends are coated. Cover hair with a plastic bag or shower cap and leave on for 30 minutes. Rinse hair well and shampoo as usual. Repeat treatment as needed.

Yield: 2 ounces, enough for 1 treatment

Banana Hair Conditioner

1 mashed banana
1 tablespoon honey

Bananas and honey make excellent conditioners for dry, sun-damaged hair because they are both rich in potassium and vitamins A, B, and C. These essential elements help to replenish lost moisture and shine. This conditioner coats the hair cuticles, leaving hair healthy and manageable. During the summer I like to use this recipe every week.

Mix together the banana and honey until smooth and creamy. Wet your hair with warm water and massage the conditioner into your hair and scalp. Wrap your hair in plastic wrap or use a towel around your head, and let the mixture condition your hair for 20 minutes. Rinse your hair well, and shampoo and condition as usual. You will notice that your hair seems thicker and your shampoo will really lather.

Yield: 2–3 ounces, enough for 1 treatment

REUNION BASKET

Summer is a popular time for reunions. Make up a basket filled with memorabilia for a special friend or family member. Use colors that represent the school, or colors of that era; for example, hot pink and lime green were popular in the seventies. Use a copy machine to make your own labels or wrapping paper from old news clippings or photographs. Because music is also a great way to remember a special time, make a tape for the intended recipient. Library reference desks have wonderful books that document what movies, books, films, and music were popular in a particular year. Have fun remembering and think of this gift as a "beauty time capsule."

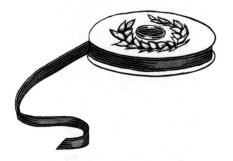

Suggested items to include:

French green clay mask (page 109)
Foaming Bath Salts in nostalgic colors
(page 225)
Banana Hair Conditioner (page 172)
Bobby pins, rollers, juice cans for setting hair
Old photos and music

If I were making up a basket for some of my college girlfriends, I would include some of the

(continued)

beauty products we used: cold cream, avocados, blue nail polish, strawberry cologne,
green clay facial masks, pink bath salts, sponge
rollers, and plastic wrap—plus plenty of old
photos that would make us all laugh.

West Indies Conditioner

1 ripe avocado, mashed
2 tablespoons sour cream or yogurt
Juice of ½ lemon (optional)

The West Indies is a large group of islands in the Caribbean Sea near South America. Several of the islands were discovered by Christopher Columbus in 1492. Avocados are just one of the many tropical fruits that grow in abundance on these islands. Local women use this hair conditioner to restore moisture and luster to their hair. If you have dry or color-treated hair, omit the lemon juice.

Mix together all ingredients and blend into a smooth paste. Massage the mixture into your hair and scalp, then wrap your hair in a warm towel or plastic shower cap and let the mixture soak into your hair for 20 minutes. Rinse well with warm water, and shampoo and style as usual.

Yield: 2 ounces, enough for 1 treatment

Lavender Hair Conditioner

This hair-strengthening recipe makes use of the stems and leaves of the lavender plant, which would otherwise be discarded. Fragrant lavender oil helps deep-condition hair, giving it luster and shine; it also helps control dandruff. The mild, pleasant scent is also very relaxing.

½ cup fresh lavender leaves and stems, cut into small pieces (I use small garden scissors to cut up the stems.)

¼ cup sunflower oil—enough to cover stems and leaves

Place the lavender leaves and stems in a small oven-proof container and cover with oil. Gently heat the mixture for 1 minute in the microwave or in a water bath. Allow the mixture to sit for at least 1 day, then strain the oil into a clean container. It will be a soft shade of green and smell faintly of lavender.

To use: Wet hair with warm water and massage approximately 1 tablespoon of the lavender oil into your hair and scalp. Wrap your hair with plastic—I find the plastic produce bags from the grocery store fit perfectly—and with a towel, turban-style. Let the mixture sit for 20–30 minutes, then shampoo as usual. Store any leftover oil in a cool, dark, dry place.

Yield: 2 ounces, enough for 4 treatments

Botanical Shampoos

Certain herbs when added to your favorite shampoo can bring out your hair's natural highlights. Chamomile makes a mild shampoo that is perfect for fine light-brown or blond hair; calendula flower petals work well for redheads; rosemary and sage are perfect for brunettes.

½ cup water

2 tablespoons dried herbs or ⅓ cup fresh

½ cup inexpensive shampoo

2 tablespoons glycerin

Mix together the water and herbs and heat gently to make a strong tea. Let the mixture steep for at least 20 minutes, then add the shampoo and glycerin, and stir well. Pour the shampoo into a clean squeeze bottle or empty shampoo bottle and let sit overnight to thicken. Shampoo as you would normally and rinse well.

Yield: 8 ounces

Natural Hair Rinses

½ cup apple cider vinegar
½ cup chopped fresh mint
1 tablespoon chopped fresh lavender
   leaves and flowers
1 cup water

Natural hair rinses are simple to create and fun to use. They serve a variety of practical purposes, such as treating dandruff, adding color, and restoring body to dull hair. They also help cleanse the scalp and promote new hair growth. Here are a few of my favorite after-shampoo hair rinse recipes.

Mix together all the ingredients and let sit overnight. Strain before using. To use, simply pour over your wet, clean hair, massage well into your scalp, then rinse with warm or cool water.

For Color:

Blondes: ¼ cup strong chamomile tea or juice of 1 lemon and 1 cup water

Redheads: ¼ cup strong red hibiscus tea

Brunettes: ¼ cup strong sage or rosemary tea

For Shine:

   1 tablespoon baking soda mixed with 1 cup water or
   ¼ cup apple cider vinegar and 1 cup water

Yield: each recipe makes enough for 1 rinse

Blackberry Leaf Hair Rinse

As summer comes to an end, one of my favorite outdoor activities is berry picking. In the Northwest, wild blackberries seem to grow everywhere—along roadsides, parks, even in backyards. Blackberries make a wonderful addition to facial masks, and you can also use them as a mild dye for dark hair. From the green prickly leaves of the blackberry bush a hair rinse can be brewed that cleanses the hair and scalp, and is a good cure for dandruff. If blackberry bushes are hard to find, look for herbal teas made from 100 percent blackberry leaves to use in this recipe.

½ cup clean fresh blackberry leaves
2 cups water

Place the leaves in a small saucepan and cover with water. Bring the water to a boil over medium heat. Lower the heat and simmer for 15 minutes. Remove the pan from the stove and allow to sit for 20 minutes. Strain the liquid and pour into a clean bottle with a stopper or lid. You will have a clear yellow-green brew with a mild berry scent.

Use as a final rinse after shampooing. For more color, add a few berries to the water before heating.

Yield: 12 ounces

CAMPGROUND BEAUTY

Summer is the perfect season for camping. Whether you are day camping or backpacking for a week, these short, simple tips will keep you looking your best in the great outdoors!

(continued)

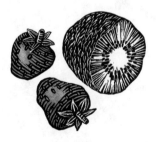

- Brush your teeth with baking soda.

- Out of mouthwash? Chewing a few juniper berries, parsley stalks, fennel seeds, or mint leaves will leave you with fresh breath.

- For a dry shampoo use cornmeal. Simply massage in and brush out.

- Need a quick pick-me-up on a hot day? Run the peel of an orange over your skin. All the essential oils are found in the peel.

- Soak your feet in a cool stream and massage with fresh peppermint leaves or peppermint oil.

- Use the abrasive strip on a matchbook for an emergency nail file.

- Tie some thyme, basil, lavender, or mint on your hat to repel flying insects.

- Soothe insect bites and bee stings with apple cider vinegar, honey, or baking soda mixed into a paste with water.

- Apply honey to any skin blemishes—it's a great spot treatment.

- Highlight your hair by rinsing it with chamomile tea or lemon juice (blonds) or rosemary tea (brunettes).

- Wild berries make nice lip stains. Mix together with a bit of petroleum jelly or aloe vera gel for a natural lipstick.

Summer Garden Cologne

This fresh, light, green cologne is perfect for summer wear. It has a mild floral scent. If you do not have fresh flowers or herbs growing in your yard, you may use the dried ingredients available at many natural food stores and farmer's markets. Because of the potency of dried ingredients, remember to use one-third the amount of the fresh ingredient called for.

2 cups vodka
Zest of 1 small lime
Zest of 1 orange
½ cup fresh lavender (petals, stems, and leaves)
½ cup fresh chamomile flower heads
¼ cup fresh chocolate mint leaves
½ cup fresh rose petals
⅛ teaspoon castor oil

Mix together all ingredients in a glass or ceramic container and cover with a lid or plastic wrap. Place in a cool, dark place and let sit for 1 week, then strain the mixture and discard all solids. Pour the cologne into a clean spray bottle or a bottle with a tight-fitting lid. If you require a stronger scent, repeat the process, adding more fresh herbs to your cologne.

Yield: 16 ounces

Cooling Cinnamon Body Powder

Try this fragrant cooling powder to soothe heat rash on a hot summer day. It contains ground cinnamon, which has a sweet, woody scent and feels great on your skin. The largest producer of cinnamon in the world is Sri Lanka, where the bark of a tropical evergreen tree in the laurel family is rolled into quills or sticks and left to dry. These dried quills are finely ground to a powder and used for a variety of purposes the world over.

½ cup cornstarch (you can also use arrowroot powder)
1 tablespoon ground cinnamon

Mix together the cornstarch and cinnamon until well blended. To use, sprinkle on skin or use a powder puff. Old spice containers make nice powder shakers.

Yield: 4¼ ounces

Sesame Oil Sunscreen

1/4 teaspoon borax powder
1/2 cup hot, strong tea (use 2 or 3
   regular tea bags, such as black
   or orange pekoe varieties, and
   strain well)
1/2 cup dark sesame oil
1 tablespoon grated beeswax

This is a recipe for a simple sunscreen that uses sesame oil and tea to help screen out the harmful rays of the sun. Sesame seed oil has one of the highest ratings for ultraviolet radiation absorption, and the tannic acid in tea also absorbs UV rays. It should be noted that this is not a sunblock, and if you have very fair skin that burns easily, use a stronger commercial sunscreen product.

Dissolve the borax in the tea, stir well, and set aside.

Mix together the oil and beeswax in a glass measuring cup, then place in a pan with about 1–2 inches of water. Heat wax and oil over medium heat on the stove top until beeswax is melted (8–10 minutes), stirring occasionally.

When the wax is melted, remove mixture from the water bath. Slowly add the tea infusion, stirring briskly. (You can also put the mixtures in the blender and blend on high speed.)

Pour the lotion into a clean container and cool completely before using. Apply to your face and body before going out in the sun, and reapply every hour during your time outdoors.

Yield: 8 ounces

SUNBURN SOOTHERS

The following list of ingredients can help take some of the stinging heat out of a bad sunburn. Remember to keep your body well hydrated by drinking plenty of water; your skin will heal faster. If you are on vacation, some of these ingredients may be available in the hotel mini-bar or from room service. Apply the ingredients directly to your skin or add to a tepid bath. Some of the soothers may dry out your skin, so use a water-based moisturizer to replenish afterward.

Sunburn-Soothing ingredients:

Vinegar (always dilute 1 tablespoon
in 1 cup of water)

Plain yogurt

Club soda

Mashed apricots

Baking soda mixed into a paste
with water

Buttermilk

Tomato juice

Witch hazel

Gin

White wine

Cucumber juice

Aloe vera gel mixed with a little vitamin E oil

Cornstarch mixed into a paste with water

Sunburn Lotion

2 tablespoons water
1 tablespoon witch hazel
¼ cup baking soda
1–2 drops peppermint oil

If you do burn easily, this simple lotion will help soothe your sensitive skin. It contains two well-known sunburn soothers — witch hazel and baking soda — along with peppermint oil, which is a natural coolant.

Mix together all the ingredients to form a thin, milky solution. Shake well before applying. To use: Gently apply to your sunburned skin and allow to dry. Reapply if necessary. You may also want to rinse your skin afterward because this lotion leaves a fine, powdery film as it dries.

Yield: 3½ ounces

Sunshine Cream

2 tablespoons liquid lecithin
¼ cup sesame oil
2 tablespoons avocado oil
¼ cup water

Sesame oil and avocado oil both have ultraviolet ray–screening properties and, when combined, make a great pre-sun skin cream. This is a mild, sunny yellow cream that I use liberally before going out in the summer. I would not recommend this cream for children or those who sunburn easily. It can be used as a moisturizing supplement to sunscreen.

Place the lecithin and oils in the blender and mix on medium speed. Slowly add the water and turn the blender on high to blend well. You will be left with a light, fluffy, yellow cream. Continue to blend on high until smooth and then place the mixture in a clean air-tight container. You may need to stir this cream every couple of days because the lecithin may separate.

Yield: 6 ounces

GROWING ALOE VERA PLANTS

For centuries aloe vera has been used around the world for the magical healing properties of the gel found within the plant's thick leaves. Cleopatra attributed her irresistible beauty to the use of aloe vera gel.

Aloe vera plants are very easy to grow and make a nice addition to your indoor (or outdoor) plant collection. The aloe family contains over two hundred different species that grow in the dry regions of Africa, Asia, Europe, and the Americas. Aloe resembles cactus in appearance but is actually a perennial succulent belonging to the lily family.

Purchase the largest plant you can find, because the potency of the gel does increase with age. The plants usually grow very slowly indoors. Aloe vera plant leaves will turn brown in harsh sunlight, so it should be kept in indirect light. It can also freeze, so it must be protected when danger of heavy frost exists. Care should be taken not to overwater the plant; it should be allowed to dry out between waterings. Be sure there is a good drainage hole in the pot so the roots don't rot. Aloe vera can stand to be root-bound, so repotting is not necessary unless the upper plant gets too "top-heavy." Mature plants will send out small shoots or "baby" plants, which can be separated and replanted. They make welcome gifts.

(continued)

Always use the leaves closest to the soil, which are larger and contain more gel. The plant grows out from the center, and cut leaves do not grow back. After cutting off the portion of the leaf you want with a sharp knife, slit the leaf lengthwise to reveal the transparent gel, which can be applied directly to the skin. If you need more gel, continue to slit the leaf until all of the gel is used and only the green skin remains. Cut leaves wrapped in plastic will keep in the refrigerator for several days. When using the gel on your skin, remember that it is naturally astringent, so be sure to moisturize well afterward. (Many commercial aloe vera products mix oil with the gel for this reason.) For a bad burn or sunburn, I like to use a bit of vitamin E oil mixed with aloe vera gel to soothe my skin.

Refreshing Travel Towels

½ cup vodka
1 teaspoon glycerin
½ cup water
10 drops lemon or orange oil
Paper towels

These cool, wet towels are perfect to take along on summer outings. Whether driving, picnicking, or camping, you'll stay clean and refreshed. They can also be used as a simple facial astringent. I package these towels in resealable plastic bags and tuck a package into my summer tote bag.

Combine all the ingredients in a small bowl. Stir to mix well.

Place folds of soft, strong paper towels together side by side in a shallow dish.

Pour the mixture over the towels and press to saturate. Stack the wet towels in a clean airtight container and cover. Repeat with more towels until the liquid is all used up. Any extra liquid can be kept in a jar with a tight-fitting lid.

Yield: up to 100 towels

NATURAL INSECT REPELLENTS

Flying and crawling pests are, unfortunately, an inevitable part of summer. But they don't necessarily have to ruin your dinner party or picnic. Several garden plants have natural insect repellents. When dining outdoors, add a few cuttings to your floral centerpiece and tie small bouquets at the legs of your table.

Citronella: One of the most popular and common natural insecticides is citronella oil. Extracted from Asiatic grass, the oil has a lemony scent that repels insects. You may purchase the essential citronella oil and add a few drops to your favorite sunscreen or lotion. I also purchased a citrosa plant at our local garden center last summer. It looks like a geranium but has the scent of citronella. Planted in a container or in the yard, the citrosa helps keep insects away.

(continued)

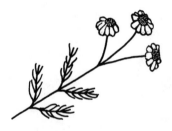

Eucalyptus: Mosquitoes do not like the scent of these fragrant trees. I like to use eucalyptus oil that is made from the leaves of the tree. I dab a small amount onto my skin and hair. Australian tea tree oil is also made from a type of eucalyptus tree. Both of these oils can be found in any natural food store. You may also use fresh leaves if you have trees growing around you. Create a strong tea by boiling up a handful of fresh leaves with some water. Spritz this scented water onto your skin and hair.

Mint: I love the scent of mint and always tuck a small bunch into my summer flower arrangements. Not only does mint provide a clean fresh scent, it helps ward off ants and flies. Basil and bay leaves work equally well.

Summer Foot Cream

¼ cup almond oil
2 tablespoons grated beeswax
2 tablespoons coconut oil
¼ cup glycerin
¼ teaspoon evening primrose oil (found at many natural food stores)
⅛ teaspoon essential oil of geranium

My girlfriend Susan gave me this summer recipe. She massages it into her feet in the evening as she watches television with her husband. This simple routine keeps her feet soft, smooth, and looking great in summer sandals!

Melt together the almond oil, beeswax, and coconut oil in a double boiler or heat-resistant glass container in the microwave.

Slowly stir in the glycerin in a thin, even stream. (I like to transfer the mixture and do this in the blender.)

Allow to cool completely and then stir in the evening primrose oil and essential oil of geranium.

Yield: 5 ounces

Foot Powder

It is important to keep your feet clean and dry during the summer months because feet confined to socks or shoes can produce more than a cup of perspiration per day! When perspiration mixes with bacteria, foot odor occurs. Rub this light powder onto your feet or sprinkle in your shoes. Your feet will stay comfortable and dry all day. The charcoal will help absorb any offending foot odor, and it's available at many health food stores. It's sometimes sold in capsule form—one capsule is approximately equal to ¼ teaspoon.

½ cup cornstarch
1 tablespoon white clay (kaolin clay)
¼ teaspoon powdered charcoal (food grade)

Mix together all the ingredients and pour into a clean, dry container. You can make a simple powder shaker by placing a piece of heavy paper over a jar, securing it with a rubber band, and poking holes in the paper with a toothpick.

Yield: 4 ounces

Tea Tree Foot Spray

Tea tree oil comes from the Australian outback and has been used by aborigines for centuries as a remedy. It is distilled from the leaves of the Australian tea tree, and it's a natural antiseptic and fungicide. It can be used at its full strength or diluted, as in this recipe. Tea tree oil makes an invigorating foot spray that can even be sprayed through nylon stockings to revive tired feet on hot days. Make sure to moisturize your feet well because the high alcohol content of the spray can dry out your skin. If you feel it's too strong or too drying, reduce the amount of vodka used.

1 teaspoon tea tree oil
¼ cup vodka
¼ cup distilled water

Mix together all the ingredients. Pour into a clean spray bottle or a container with a tight-fitting lid.

Yield: 4 ounces

Giggly Wiggly Footbath

1 box fruit-flavored gelatin; size depends on your footbath container—one 3-ounce box usually works well for my small sink basin
Warm water

This is a footbath that is both fun and relaxing. My daughter Marie loves it. She laughs and wiggles her toes the entire time. It helps clean, soften, and refresh tired feet and is especially energizing after a long hot day.

Make the gelatin according to the package directions using twice the amount of water; that is, for a 3-ounce box I use 4 cups of water.

Let the gelatin cool in the refrigerator until set. It's nice to prepare it in the morning for end-of-day baths.

To use: Pour the gelatin into your foot bath container—anything that holds water will work. Sit down and soak your feet for at least 10 minutes. Rinse well and massage with a rich foot cream.

Yield: 32 ounces, enough for 1 foot bath

THE ULTIMATE PEDICURE

The word *pedicure* means "caring for the feet," which is more than just soaking your feet and clipping your toenails. The steps that follow may take you almost an hour to complete, but the results are well worth it. It is an intense, long-lasting all-over treatment from which your whole body can benefit. It is amazing how good you feel when your feet are cared for properly. In the summer, weekly pedicures are especially important to keep feet looking and feeling their best.

(continued)

Steps to follow for healthy, happy feet:

1. Soak feet for 15–20 minutes in a warm foot-bath or salt water. Use a nail brush and really clean under each toenail. Use a wet pumice stone or exfoliating scrub to gently rub away tough skin on the soles of your feet and heels.

2. Trim your toenails *after* soaking them. It is easier to do this when your nails are soft, and you will get a cleaner cut. Cut the nails straight across to avoid ingrown toenails.

3. Put on a good foot mask. Use your favorite facial mask recipe—I like to use green clay mixed with some peppermint oil and water. Elevate your feet and leave the mask on for 15–20 minutes.

4. Place your feet back in the footbath and rinse away all of the foot mask.

5. Massage a rich cuticle cream into your toe-nails and gently push back the cuticles at the base of each nail.

6. Massage a rich cream into each foot. Wrap your feet in plastic wrap and again elevate your feet for 15–20 minutes, or slip on a pair of cotton socks.
   Note: If you are doing an evening pedicure, you may want to leave socks on all night.

Autumn Skin and Hair Care

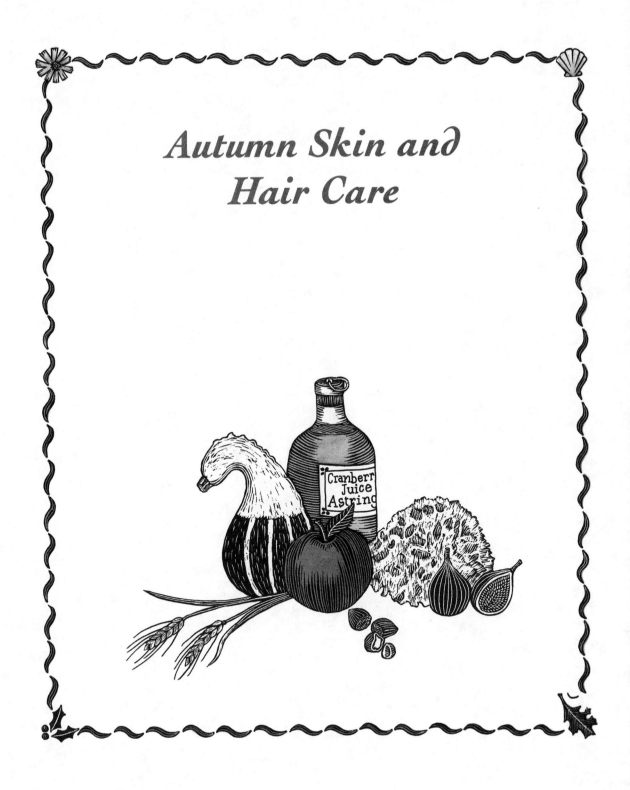

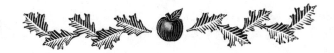

I cling to summer as long as I can, but eventually I have to admit that the long sunny days, along with my tan, are fading. During the first few weeks of October, I cut back all of my summer perennials and herbs and start decorating with pumpkins and gourds. I turn to the orchards and fields for beauty inspiration and enjoy using fresh apples, nuts, and grains in my recipes and treatments. This is a time of harvest and gathering, and beauty ingredients are no exception. Many of my favorite fresh fruits, such as fragrant quinces, ripe pears, fresh figs, and soft persimmons, make only a brief appearance at the market this time of year. I love to use the fresh quince seeds as a hair setting gel (see page 218), and this is my only chance to gather them!

Autumn is also a season of change and excitement that fosters both beginnings and endings. With the end of summer comes the start of the school year and the busy holiday season. The weather is changing to crisp, cool mornings and chilly evenings, and these conditions make for drier skin and hair. Using more oil-rich products is again important to keep your skin and hair full of moisture. The Walnut Oil Cream on page 201 is an excellent way to make use of fresh fall nuts, and it makes a super night cream! The use of a cleansing scrub such as the Hazelnut Cleansing Scrub on page 197 is also a good idea to help even out fading tans and give your skin a fresh, healthy glow.

With drier conditions both inside and out, many people (myself included) experience "fly-away" hair. Using a weekly deep-conditioning treatment will keep your hair fully hydrated and easier to manage. My favorite simple hair conditioner is honey. It does wonders for dry, damaged hair and washes out easily. Simply massage a tablespoon or two into damp hair before washing and let sit for fifteen to twenty minutes, then shampoo as usual. Honey does have mild bleaching qualities, so if you have very dark hair, you can use molasses or maple syrup.

Autumn also marks the start of a busy holiday season. Evening scents and appearances need to be more exotic and glamorous. Caramel and vanilla have become popular base note scents in fragrance products and make wonderful autumn perfumes. I have used pure vanilla extract from the bottle as an evening scent. It makes a wonderful autumn cologne, soft and sweet.

There are several wonderful holiday gifts you can make this season. Surprise a friend with a special treat on Halloween (see Happy Haunting on page 202). Or bring the whole family a basketful of bath goodies for Thanksgiving—a great way for everyone to relax after a big day.

Both of my daughters enjoy making their own gifts for the holidays. Just after Thanksgiving is when we sit down and put together our holiday gift lists. The Foaming Bath Salts (page 225) is a new twist on our favorite colored bath salts recipe and just as simple to create. We make several batches of different colors and scents for everyone on our list. (We also make an extra batch for ourselves!)

For a description of common autumn ingredients and where to find them, see page 24.

BASE NOTES

Base notes are the longer lasting fragrance elements. A base note or low note is the scent that lingers on the skin. Vanilla is a base note because it contains fixatives that give a lasting quality to the scent or ingredients it is mixed with.

Simply Natural Facial Steam Baths

A facial steam bath is an easy, inexpensive, and therapeutic way to deep-cleanse your skin. Gently steaming the skin creates perspiration, which aids in the elimination of toxins, boosts circulation, and softens the skin.

Follow this schedule for great results: For normal skin, steam weekly; oily skin, steam twice weekly; dry skin, every other week. Do not use a facial steam if you have a serious skin problem without checking first with your physician.

Using dried herbs in your facial benefits your skin by boosting circulation and enhancing the cleansing effects of the steam. I have listed a few common herbs to try:

For oily skin: calendula, geranium, sage, and yarrow

For dry skin: parsley, fennel, chamomile, and lemon verbena

For normal skin: rose petals, mint, thyme, chervil, and lavender

3 tablespoons dried herbs
6 cups boiling water

Secure your hair and cleanse your face as you would normally. Place the dried herbs in a large ceramic bowl. Pour boiling water over the herbs and stir. Keep your face at least 12 inches away and use a large bath towel to make a tent over your head and the bowl. Close your eyes and steam for 10–15 minutes. Rinse your face with warm and then cool water, and gently pat your skin dry. Your skin is sensitive after a facial, so stay indoors for at least 1 hour after treatment to allow your pores to close completely.

Yield: 1 treatment

Harvest Maiden Scrubs

My father was a barley farmer, and harvest time was very important to our family. After a summer of caring for the crop, autumn was a time of hard work and excitement. Today, I celebrate those times by making up jars of fresh cleansing grains to use throughout the year and give as gifts. Barley and other natural grains make excellent face and body scrubs for all skin types. For gift-giving, cover your jar lid with some natural textured fabric and attach a few sheaves of wheat or barley.

Oatmeal: This popular grain is a beauty pantry staple. It works well for all skin types and can be used to cleanse the skin in place of soap and water. Whole-grain oatmeal cereal is more effective than the more expensive quick-cooking versions.

Wheat germ: Wheat germ is very high in protein and vitamins E and B. Because of its soothing and healing properties, wheat germ makes a gentle facial scrub that is perfect for sensitive and dry skin.

Barley: Fresh barley is an age-old skin beautifier that makes a gentle scrub to soothe and smooth rough skin. Many natural food stores now stock a wide variety of grains, including barley.

Semolina flour: Italians will tell you the importance of semolina flour for their hearty pasta diet. Made from durum wheat, it is used to make pasta dough. Because it is a coarse flour, semolina also makes an excellent skin exfoliator. The flour comes ready to use from the sack and can be found at the grocery store in the flour aisle, sometimes labeled "pasta flour."

Select one or several of the grains listed. Using a spice or coffee grinder, coarsely grind 1 or 2 tablespoons of the grains until they become flourlike, then pour into a clean jar. To use: Combine 1–2 teaspoons of the mixture with equal parts water or cleanser to create a thick, smooth paste. You will need more if you are doing your whole body (approximately ½ cup). Massage this paste gently into your skin, rinse well with tepid water, and pat dry.

Yield: 2 to 4 ounces (depending on the amount of grains used)

Hazelnuts—or filberts, as they're sometimes called—are native to the state of Oregon where they grow in such abundance that they provide for 98 percent of the nation's supply. These nuts are harvested in October and are rich in natural oils that keep your skin soft and radiant. They have a long shelf life and can stay fresh up to a year if kept in a sealed bag at room temperature, and longer if stored in the freezer.

Mix all the ingredients together. Store in a clean container. To use: Massage into face and neck. The scrub will seem a bit rough because of the ground hazelnuts. Rinse well with tepid water and pat dry.

Yield: 2 ounces

Hazelnut Cleansing Scrub

1 tablespoon finely ground hazelnuts
1 tablespoon cleansing lotion or cold cream
1 teaspoon honey

Brown Sugar Cleanser

Soap and water
1 teaspoon dark brown sugar

Dark brown sugar makes a good abrasive skin scrub when combined with your regular soap or facial wash. It dissolves gently and is fine enough to be used on the face. You can also scrub your whole body with brown sugar—you'll feel clean and stimulated. If you wish, white sugar may also be used in this recipe.

While washing your face with soap, add a teaspoon of dark brown sugar to the lather and massage gently into your skin. Rinse your skin with warm water followed by a splash of cold water. Pat dry.

Yield: enough for 1 facial cleansing

Cranberry Juice Astringent

¼ cup pure cranberry juice
2 tablespoons vodka
2 tablespoons witch hazel

Cranberry harvest begins about the third week of September and peaks in mid-October; the crisp, cool autumn days make great weather for berry harvesting. These bright red cranberries make a wonderful simple facial mask that gives a rosy glow to your skin. The acidity in the cranberries works as a mild astringent and leaves my skin sparkling clean. It works well for all skin types.

Mix all the ingredients together. Bottle in an airtight container. Apply to your skin using a clean cotton ball.

Yield: 4 ounces

Apple Pectin Toner

For centuries, apples have been an integral part of our lives as a basic food source and beauty ingredient. Apples are 85 percent water and high in vitamins A and C, and potassium, but their seeds contain toxins and should always be removed. *Apple pectin is a natural thickener and is often used in recipes as an alternative to gelatin. When applied as a facial toner, pectin is soothing and refreshing for all skin types.*

Place the cut-up apple in a small saucepan with the water. Bring to a boil and remove from the heat. Allow the mixture to cool completely, then strain out the apple chunks. Stir in the witch hazel and pour into a clean container. To use: Spray or apply to skin using a clean cotton ball.

Yield: 6 ounces

1 apple, cut up with peel, seeds removed (The color of the peel will give the toner a hint of color; red apples create a pretty pink toner.)
½ cup water
¼ cup witch hazel

Rose Hip Skin Tonic

This simple rose-colored tea made from fresh or dried rose hips is loaded with vitamin C and acts as a sublime tonic for a dull, lifeless complexion. Dried rose hips and rose hip powder can be found at many natural food stores and make a flavorful addition to morning teas and juices. Women in Scandinavia use rose hip tea to improve their complexions and enhance their natural beauty from the inside out.

In a small ceramic bowl or cup, place the dried rose hips or rose hip powder. Pour the boiling water over the rose hips and allow the mixture to steep for 15 minutes, then strain the mixture and allow to cool com-

1 tablespoon dried rose hips or rose hip powder
1 cup boiling water
1 tablespoon witch hazel

pletely. Add the witch hazel and pour into a clean container. Apply to just-washed skin using a clean cotton ball or pad.

Yield: 8 ounces

Gourmet Hand Cream

2 tablespoons olive oil
2 teaspoons honey
1 teaspoon liquid lecithin
½ teaspoon apple cider vinegar

Many professional chefs rub olive oil into their hands before starting to cook. Because they are constantly washed and dried, a cook's hands need to be moisturized frequently. This is an excellent cream to whip up before creating your next gourmet meal. It also makes a welcome gift for someone who loves to cook and whose hands show it! I keep a small jar next to my kitchen sink. Because the ingredients are all edible, you can have this cream on your hands when preparing food.

In the blender or with a wire whisk, mix all the ingredients together until well combined. Pour into a clean container with a tight-fitting lid. It may seem a bit sticky at first, but this stickiness will go away after sitting for a day or two.

Yield: 3 ounces

Tahitian Scented Coconut Oil

Tahiti's national flower is the fragrant, white, star-shaped Gardenia Taitensis and is honored in a fete each year celebrated during the first week of December. Scented coconut oil, made by placing dried gardenia flowers inside bottles of pure coconut oil, is a popular beauty product used as a tanning oil (it contains no sunscreen), skin moisturizer, and hair conditioner. Even if you do not have access to Tahitian gardenias, you can make your own scented oil using gardenia flower fragrance oil or extract.

2–3 drops gardenia fragrance or oil
1 dried gardenia flower (optional)
½ cup coconut oil

In a clean glass jar or bottle, place 1 dried gardenia flower and several drops of gardenia fragrance.

Gently warm the coconut oil until it becomes liquid. This can be done by placing it in a warm place or allowing the oil container to sit in a pan of hot water.

Pour the melted coconut oil into the container and allow to sit for 1 week in a dark, dry place.

Yield: 4 ounces

Walnut Oil Cream

Walnut trees have been cultivated in Europe since Roman times for both culinary and cosmetic use. The oil extracted from the walnut contains essential fatty acids important for maintaining beautiful skin and hair. This rich cream can be massaged into dry hands, and a tablespoon mixed with vitamin E oil produces a remarkable eye cream. I find walnut oil in the cooking oil section of my local grocery store.

2 tablespoons grated beeswax
¼ cup coconut oil
¼ cup walnut oil
2 tablespoons rosewater

In a heat-resistant container, mix together the beeswax and oils. Heat gently in the microwave or a water bath until the wax and coconut oil are melted. Stir in the rosewater and pour into a clean container. You may have to stir once or twice to keep the oil and water blended as the mixture cools into a thick cream.

Yield: 4 ounces

HAPPY HAUNTING

Make up a Halloween basket for your favorite ghoul friend that's guaranteed to raise his or her spirits. In it, place a small jar of French green clay, a jar of Walnut Oil Cream (page 201), and scented theme soaps shaped like bats, ghosts, and spiders (see the recipe for Simple Fancy Soaps on page 235). Fill clear plastic gloves (available at restaurant supply shops) with cleansing grains or colored bath salts and tie the wrists closed with colored ribbons. Trick or treat!

Evening Repair Lotion

¼ teaspoon baking soda
½ cup distilled water
1 tablespoon vitamin E oil
2 tablespoons almond oil
1 tablespoon walnut or hazelnut oil
¼ teaspoon wheat germ oil
½ teaspoon honey
1 tablespoon grated beeswax

After a day spent outside in crisp, dry autumn weather, you'll need to use this rich lotion in the evening before going to bed to restore lost moisture to your skin. You'll wake up in the morning to soft, smooth skin. You can also use this lotion during the day as a rich moisturizer or eye cream. Use only a small amount on your skin because it is extremely rich in natural oils. All the oils listed should be easily found at the grocery store or natural food store.

Dissolve the baking soda with the water in a glass measuring cup and set aside.

Mix together the oils, honey, and beeswax in

another glass measuring cup. Place the oil mixture in a pan of water (about 1–2 inches), making a water bath. Heat the oil mixture in the water bath over medium heat until the beeswax is melted (8–10 minutes), stirring occasionally.

When the wax is melted, heat the soda-water mixture to near boiling. This can be done in the microwave (on High for 1 minute) or in the same water bath you used to heat the oil mixture.

Remove the oil mixture from the heat and slowly add it to the water solution, stirring briskly. (You can also place in the blender and whip.)

Pour the lotion into a clean container with a lid. The lotion will thicken as it cools. Apply over your body after it has cooled completely.

Yield: 6 ounces

Mashed Potato Hand Cream

Raw potato is an old and very effective folk remedy used to treat eczema, or dry, flaky skin. When my grandmother was a child, slices of fresh potato were rubbed over the body as a moisturizer. In this recipe, mashed potatoes make up a rich moisturizing hand cream. I find this cream a bit sticky for daytime use. You may want to rinse after using it or massage into your hands in the evening and cover with cotton or plastic gloves.

Blend together all the ingredients into a smooth, thick paste. To use: Massage a small amount into your hands. After 5–10 minutes, rinse hands.

Yield: 4 ounces

2 medium-size potatoes, peeled, cooked, and mashed
1 tablespoon glycerin
1 tablespoon potato water
1 tablespoon light oil

Tapioca Facial Mask

1 tablespoon small-pearl tapioca
2 tablespoons water

Tapioca is a popular food starch that comes from the root of the tropical cassava plant. The dried starchy granules extracted from the root are called "pearls." This is the form you will find tapioca in at your grocery store. They need to be soaked for at least one hour before being used. Instant tapioca can also be used in this recipe. Because the granules are finer, instant tapioca does not need to be soaked for quite as long. This simple facial mask leaves your skin soft and smooth, and works for all skin types.

Mix together the tapioca and water, and let sit overnight or for several hours until soft. (This is the required soaking mentioned above.) With the back of a spoon or fork, mix the soft tapioca until you have a smooth paste. Massage this paste into your face and neck, and let sit for 10–15 minutes until dry. Rinse with warm water.

Yield: 2 ounces, enough for 1 mask

Fig Facial Mask

One fresh, ripe fig

My grandmother used to have a fig tree in her backyard. My sister and I loved to pick and eat the sweet fruits whenever we visited her. Fresh figs make a splendid facial mask. They contain a special protein-tenderizing substance, as do papaya and pineapples, which helps to rid skin of surface impurities and dead skin cells. Many people also feel it helps to reduce fine lines and wrinkles, making the skin appear smoother. Because of their high enzyme content, they should remain on your skin only a short period of time—no more than five minutes. Fresh figs are extremely perishable and should be used right away. *Dried figs can also be used but should be soaked for about fifteen minutes in water or apple juice until they are plump and soft.*

Slice the fig in half and turn each half inside out to reveal the soft interior. Scrape the inside flesh into a bowl and mash with the back of a fork until smooth. Spread the mixture onto clean skin and let sit for 5 minutes. Rinse with warm water followed by cool water and moisturize your skin.

Yield: approximately 2 ounces, enough for 1 facial mask

Artichoke Facial Mask

Artichokes were first grown near the Mediterranean Sea. Here in the United States, most of the ones we see in the markets are from California. These large thistlelike plants produce an edible flower bud that contains a number of vitamins and minerals, including vitamin A and potassium. The interior of these buds is called the "heart" and is a true beauty delicacy. Artichoke hearts make a wonderful facial mask. I like to use avocado oil in this recipe, but any light oil will leave your skin looking radiant.

1 fresh artichoke heart, well cooked, or canned hearts in water, not oil
2 teaspoons light oil (avocado, olive, canola)
½ teaspoon vinegar or fresh lemon juice

In a small ceramic bowl, mash the artichoke heart and mix in the oil and vinegar. Stir well, until you have a smooth paste. Massage the mixture onto your face and neck, and let sit for 10–15 minutes. Rinse off with warm water and pat your skin dry.

Yield: 1 treatment

Persimmon Facial Mask

½ fresh, ripe persimmon, peel and all

Common persimmons are grown primarily in the southeastern states, such as South Carolina and Florida. They are particularly abundant in the autumn months. These bright orange, pulpy fruits taste best when almost overripe. Persimmons contain the same acid level as normal, healthy skin and make an ideal facial mask for deep-cleaning all types of skin.

Mash the persimmon into a smooth consistency. Spread the mixture over your clean face and neck. Allow it to dry for 10 minutes or longer and then wash off with warm water. For oily skin, mash the pulp and use it mixed with a little cornstarch or egg white. For extra-dry skin, mix with an egg yolk and 1–2 teaspoons of almond oil.

Yield: approximately 2 ounces, enough for 1 mask

Russian Rose Hip Facial Mask

20 fresh or dried rose hips
½ cup water

The fruit of the rose is the rose hip. They are picked in the late fall, just before the frost destroys them, and can be eaten in soups, teas, and jellies. They also make wonderful beauty products. The Russians call them "vitamin roses" since they contain more vitamin C than any other known natural source (forty times more than oranges). They are also rich in calcium, iron, and vitamin A. If you cannot pick fresh rose hips, dried ones are available at most natural food stores.

Remove the stalks and blossom ends of the rose hips. Wash in cold water. Cut or break the rose hips in half and remove the seeds and "hair" from the shells with your fingers. Place in a small saucepan and cover with the water. Bring the mixture to a boil and simmer for 10–15 minutes. (If you are using dried rose hips, let them soak in the water overnight to soften before simmering.) Pour the cooked mixture into a blender or food processor and process until you have a smooth puree. Let cool, then apply to your skin and allow to sit for 10–15 minutes. Rinse with cool water and pat dry. Any leftover mask should be stored in the refrigerator.

Yield: approximately 6 ounces

Pear Ambrosia Facial Mask

I live in Oregon's Rogue Valley where fresh pears mark the arrival of autumn. They are an excellent source of sorbitol, a natural sugar substitute and humectant that moisturizes and softens your skin. Ambrosial means "worthy of the gods," and this treatment is. This mask is especially soothing if your skin is sun- or wind-damaged, or if you have unsightly blotches or redness.

1 fresh, ripe pear
½ teaspoon honey
1 tablespoon heavy cream

Peel and core the pear. Cut up into small pieces and place in a small dish. With a fork, mash the fruit into a smooth paste. Add the honey and cream. Using a small pastry brush or your fingers, spread the mixture evenly over your face and neck. Let sit for 15 minutes and then rinse with warm water. Splash your face with cool water and pat dry.

Yield: 3–4 ounces, enough for 1 mask

THE PERFECT FACIAL

Skin cells regenerate every twenty-one days, so a monthly facial is essential for maintaining a healthy and glowing complexion. A complete facial involves a six-step process: analyzing, steaming, massaging the skin, applying the mask, rinsing the face, and moisturizing the skin with a strong protective cream. Facials may take up to an hour to complete, but they're worth the effort. Not only your skin but your whole body will feel refreshed and clean.

Six steps to beautiful skin:

1. **Analyze:** Gently wash your face with a mild cleanser and pat dry. Pull your hair back from your face and secure. Examine your skin carefully in the mirror using a good strong light. Is it dry, oily? Take note of blackheads or blemishes and pluck any stray facial hair with tweezers.

2. **Steam:** Fill your bathroom sink with hot water, then make a tent with a towel and lean forward over the basin. Let the steam envelop your face for 5–10 minutes. Steam baths help soften the skin, opening pores and extracting impurities. Adding a few drops of essential oil to the hot water will enhance your steam "session." I love lavender's soothing fragrance.

(continued)

Note: If you have severe acne, skip this step. Steaming is not recommended for badly broken-out skin, since it can aggravate the condition by stimulating blood vessels and activating oil glands.

3. **Massage:** Using your fingertips, gently massage your face in smooth upward strokes. The length of the facial massage depends on your skin type: twelve to fifteen minutes for dry skin and as little as five minutes for oily skin, to avoid producing more oil.

4. **Facial mask:** This is the most relaxing part of the facial process. Create a fresh mask based on your skin analysis: for dry skin, a moisturizing mask containing egg yolk or banana; for oily skin, an astringent mask using egg whites or aloe vera gel. Using your fingers or a small pastry brush, spread the mask onto your face and neck. Create a thin even layer, avoiding the delicate skin around your eyes. Leave the mask on for fifteen to twenty minutes to dry thoroughly.

5. **Rinse:** Rinse your face with warm water. Follow with a cool-water rinse for at least one minute, then pat your skin dry.

6. **Moisturize:** Using your favorite facial moisturizer, massage the cream or lotion onto your face and neck, and allow it to soak in. Your skin will look radiant, and your body will feel recuperated and revitalized.

Whipped Cream Body Mask

1 cup fresh heavy cream

In 1965, my parents bought the album Whipped Cream & Other Delights *by Herb Alpert and the Tijuana Brass. I remember so many of the songs from it: "A Taste of Honey," "Tangerine," "Love Potion Number 9," and "Whipped Cream" were some of my favorites. But it was the album jacket that caught my eye. On it was a beautiful woman covered in whipped cream. It was a beauty fantasy too good to be true! As it turns out, fresh cream is extremely beneficial to the skin because it contains protein and lactic acid, which help soften and nourish the skin. This treatment feels wonderful, especially with Herb Alpert playing in the background.*

Using an electric mixer or a wire whisk and a large bowl, whip the fresh cream until soft peaks form and you have a soft, fluffy consistency. To use: Slather the cream all over the body, including your hair if you wish, and massage well. Leave the mixture on for 5–10 minutes; you may wrap yourself up in a large towel and lie down. Rinse off in a warm bath or shower and pat your skin dry.

Yield: 8 ounces, enough for 1 whole body treatment

Cranberry Lip Gloss

1 tablespoon almond oil
10 fresh cranberries
1 teaspoon honey

Fresh cranberries give this simple gloss a hint of color and natural flavor. I enjoy this sweet gloss as is, but if you prefer more shine, you can mix one teaspoon of petroleum jelly into the finished product.

Mix together all the ingredients and place them in a microwave or heat-resistant container. Heat in the microwave or a water bath until the mixture just begins to boil (1–2 minutes in the microwave). Stir well and gently mash the berries. Let sit for 5 minutes. Strain the mixture through a fine sieve to remove all pieces of cranberry. Stir and allow to cool completely. When cool, spoon into a clean container. To use: Simply spread a small amount onto your lips.

Yield: ½ ounce

Canola Oil Lip Balm

1 teaspoon canola oil
1 teaspoon castor oil
1 teaspoon grated beeswax

Canola oil is a popular cooking oil easily found at the grocery store. It is an occlusive oil, which means it increases the water content of the skin and lips by sealing the surface and holding moisture in. You can also use this recipe on your eyebrows to condition them and keep them neat.

Melt together the oils and beeswax in a glass measuring cup in a pan of boiling water over medium heat (water bath technique). Pour the melted mixture into a lip gloss container or other small, clean container and allow to cool completely, approximately 20 minutes. To use: Spread a small amount onto your lips.

Yield: ½ ounce

Vanilla Lip Gloss

1 tablespoon grated beeswax
½ tablespoon coconut oil
⅛ teaspoon vitamin E oil
⅛ teaspoon vanilla extract

Last year my mother-in-law brought me a wonderful vanilla extract from Mexico, where some of the finest vanilla in the world is produced. Vanilla extract gives this lip gloss a lovely scent and caramel color, not to mention delectable vanilla flavor. This lip gloss recipe smells good enough to eat!

Place the beeswax, coconut oil, and vitamin E oil in an ovenproof container. Heat gently until the wax and oils are melted. Stir in the vanilla extract and mix well. Pour the mixture into a clean container and allow to cool completely.

Yield: ¾ ounce

Apple Juice Mouth Rinse

½ cup fresh apple juice
1 tablespoon rosewater
Pinch of dried mint, ginger, or
    cinnamon (optional)

An apple a day will keep the doctor away—and your mouth feeling fresh and clean. Unsweetened apple juice makes a good, simple mouth rinse. Dried mint, ginger, and cinnamon can also be added to this recipe. All are naturally antiseptic and add a mildly sweet flavor to the rinse.

Mix together all ingredients in a clean container and shake gently to mix. To use: Rinse a teaspoon or two through the mouth.

Yield: 4 ounces

Clear Mascara

1 tablespoon castor oil

Castor oil is made from the seed of the castor plant. This pale, unscented oil makes an excellent conditioner for your eyelashes and eyebrows. It gives them healthy, protective shine and can be used in place of colored mascara for a more natural look that won't leave black rings under your eyes. Castor oil is usually found in the health-care section of the grocery store or at the pharmacy.

Pour the castor oil into a small bottle. Using a clean mascara brush, apply a small amount of oil to clean, dry lashes. I save the brushes from old mascara containers and soak them in a mild detergent until they are clean, then let air-dry.

Yield: ½ ounce

Potato Flour Shampoo

¼ cup potato flour
2 cups water
2 teaspoons apple cider vinegar

Potato flour or potato starch is a flour made from potatoes, ground to a pulp and washed of all fibers. It swells in hot water to form a thick, creamy gel. In this recipe it is used to make a gentle nonsoap shampoo that is excellent for extremely dry hair.

Combine the flour and water in a saucepan using a wire whisk until the mixture is smooth and creamy. (I sometimes mix the flour and water in a blender and then pour it into the saucepan.)

Gently warm the mixture on low heat for 20 minutes—but do not boil. Remove from the heat and stir in the vinegar. Let the shampoo cool completely, then pour into a clean container. Use as you would any shampoo product.

Yield: 12 ounces

Molasses and Apple Cider Hair Conditioner

1 teaspoon walnut oil
1 teaspoon canola oil
1 teaspoon olive oil
1 egg yolk
1 tablespoon molasses
1 tablespoon apple cider vinegar

The crisp, cooler days of autumn can cause your hair to become dry and brittle. This oil-rich conditioner contains molasses, which, like honey, is a natural humectant. This recipe will keep your hair soft, radiant, and full of moisture. And don't worry—the molasses will easily rinse right out when you shampoo your hair.

Mix together all the ingredients, stirring thoroughly.

Massage into your hair and scalp. Wrap your hair in plastic wrap or use a plastic shower cap and leave the conditioner on your hair for 15 minutes.

Shampoo your hair as usual and rinse well. Finish with a cool water rinse.

Yield: 2 ounces, enough for 1 treatment

Ginger Hair Oil

1 teaspoon grated fresh gingerroot
¼ cup light sesame oil

This treatment is very effective in stimulating hair growth. It also helps alleviate dandruff and boosts your scalp's circulation. I would not recommend this oil for sensitive skin types because the ginger is spicy and may irritate sensitive scalps. This recipe will leave your hair smelling faintly of ginger—a scent I happen to like, especially in the fall.

Place the grated ginger inside a piece of cheesecloth and gently squeeze ¼ teaspoon of the juice into the sesame oil. Mix the oil and juice together with a fork or small whisk until well blended. To use: Massage the oil into your scalp and leave on for 10 minutes before shampooing. This oil may also be left on the head as a pack treatment, but if your scalp is irritated by the ginger, wash your hair at once and reduce the amount of ginger used.

Yield: 2 ounces

Saxon Hair Dyes

The Saxons were a hardy Germanic tribe who invaded the island of Britain twenty-five hundred years ago. Before going into battle they would often dye their hair vivid shades of green, blue, and orange to give themselves a psychological edge. You do not necessarily have to achieve the drastic results that the Saxons desired, but by using natural ingredients you can create bright highlights in your own hair and give yourself a boost! It is important to always do a swatch test first to establish the shade you are trying to achieve.

½ cup pure henna powder, your choice of color (You may need to use more powder if you have very long hair.)

¼ cup boiling distilled water (Chlorine in tap water can cause color to change.)

FACE AND SCALP TREAT

Double up treatments in one twenty-minute beauty session. Wash your face and dampen your hair, then apply a deep-cleansing clay mask. While it dries, stimulate your scalp with a dab of essential oil—I like to use rosemary. Work the pads of your fingers in tiny circles from the center of your forehead to the nape of your neck, then from your temples to the nape of your neck, and end by massaging from the region below your ears to the nape of your neck.

Henna provides the most consistent results using natural ingredients. It is also the easiest dye to find and use. Most people think of henna for creating red hair shades, but in fact it can be used on all colors from blond to black, to either enhance or change your own natural color. Henna color will last in your hair for three to six months. Henna gradually washes out, so you will not have "dark" roots.

To dye hair with natural henna: Decide on the shade you would like to have. Remember that you cannot go lighter with henna. You can condition light hair with neutral henna. Henna comes in such shades as strawberry, auburn, red, light brown, brown, dark brown, and black. Many natural food and health food stores sell it in bulk or in kit form.

Place the henna powder in a ceramic, glass, or plastic container and slowly add the boiling water, stirring until you have a paste the consistency of mud. You may need to add a little more water.

Using protective gloves (so that you do not dye your hands) apply the henna to clean, dry hair. Cover your entire head with the henna and massage well into your hair, through to the ends. Wrap your hair in plastic wrap or use a plastic shower cap.

Keep your head warm: Sit in the sun, use a handheld blow-dryer, or sit under a warm hair dryer. I like to wrap a warm towel over my head, turban-style. Do this for 15 to 45 minutes. The longer the henna is left on your hair, the darker the color will become. Rinse your hair thoroughly with warm water until the water runs clear. Shampoo your hair and rinse well.

Some variations to try:

TO HIGHLIGHT BLOND HAIR: Substitute strong chamomile tea for the water and use neutral-colored henna.

FOR COPPER AND GOLDEN HIGHLIGHTS IN BROWN HAIR: Add 3 tablespoons lemon juice to the boiling water and use brown henna.

FOR DARKER BROWN TONES: Use strong coffee or espresso in place of water and use dark brown or black henna.

FOR RED HIGHLIGHTS: Add 1 teaspoon paprika to the boiling water and use auburn or red henna.

FOR EXTRA CONDITIONING: Add 1 egg to the henna mixture or 1 tablespoon light oil.

Yield: enough for 1 treatment

Black Velvet Hair Rinse

A Black Velvet is a popular English drink, but few people realize that it also makes a great finishing hair rinse and will give your hair extra body and bounce. Don't worry if the spirits have gone flat; the alcohol's effect will leave your hair feeling healthy and vibrant.

½ cup champagne
½ cup stout beer

Mix together the champagne and stout beer. Pour the mixture over just-shampooed hair and style as usual. Any extra beer or champagne may be kept in the refrigerator for other rinses.

Yield: 8 ounces, enough for 1 rinse

Quince Seed Setting Gel

Seeds from 1 fresh quince
    (20–25 seeds)
¼ cup water

Quinces are fragrant, fuzzy fruits that appear to be a cross between an apple and a pear. Yet they actually belong to the rose family. Quinces are very bitter and because of this are almost never eaten fresh. Many seeds can be found inside the fruit's core, and when soaked in water, they make an excellent hair-setting gel.

Place the seeds in a glass or ceramic container. Pour the water over the seeds and allow the mixture to sit for several hours. The quince seeds will give off a clear, gel-like liquid. The longer the seeds sit, the thicker the mixture will become—I usually let it sit overnight. To use: Before styling your hair, work a small amount of the setting gel into it as you would any styling gel. You can also spray the liquid onto your hair.

Yield: 2 ounces

DECORATED HAIR ACCESSORIES

Now that the colder weather is back and people let their hair grow out, I like to dress up plain hair accessories to give as gifts. Here are a few of my favorite ideas. You may give them alone or tuck them into a gift basket with some Molasses and Apple Cider Hair Conditioner (page 214) or some Quince Seed Setting Gel (above).

(continued)

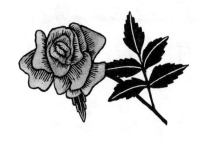

Decoupage: This easy Victorian craft is as popular today as ever. Decorate barrettes, wooden brushes, and combs with pretty "scraps" of paper. I like to cut out magazine photos and funny sayings to create unique hair brushes that bring a smile when used. There are many good decoupage finishes available today at craft stores. White glue can also be used, thinned with a bit of water. After two or three coats, follow up with a layer of paste wax for a waterproof finish.

Paint: Give plain wooden combs and brushes a fresh new look with water-based acrylic paints. Draw a design or create dots, stripes, or flowers in bright colors. Apply a final protective coat of clear varnish.

Pressed flowers: You can press pretty flowers, leaves, even seaweed to enhance any accessory. Simply place your object, the leaves or petals, carefully between pieces of wax paper and tuck inside a heavy book. When dry, they can be glued onto combs and brushes and coated with a layer of varnish. Follow up with a coat of paste wax, and you've made a lasting beauty heirloom.

Old-Fashioned Beauty Bath

1 cup barley
1 cup bran
1 cup oatmeal
1 cup brown rice
¼ cup dried bay leaves
¼ cup dried lavender flowers
4 quarts fresh rainwater (This was
    easier in my grandmother's
    time—today, tap water will do.)

This is an old-time recipe my grandmother used for decades—she got it from her mother! It uses a combination of grains and fragrant herbs for a really relaxing bath treatment. The grains help soften your bathwater and make your skin feel as smooth as silk. Follow up with a vigorous towel drying, and your skin will practically glow with health.

Place all the ingredients in a large saucepan. Bring the mixture to a boil, then lower the heat and simmer for 1 hour. Strain the mixture, removing all solids. Pour half of the liquid into a tub of bathwater. Reserve the other half for another bath or give to a friend. Store in the refrigerator.

Yield: enough for 2 baths

Vin Aigre Bath

1 cup sour wine or wine vinegar

*V*in aigre *is French for sour wine. Using wine and wine vinegars in the bath to soften the skin and restore its natural acid balance is a technique used by beautiful women for centuries. Both Helen of Troy and Mary Queen of Scots bathed regularly in wine and wine vinegar. I prefer red wine vinegars, as they give the bath a rosy color, but white wine works equally well. Save any wine left over from your table and allow it to "sour" (let it sit unopened at room temperature for several days). Tied up with a satin bow, this is a perfect last-minute gift to bring to a dinner party.*

Pour the *vin aigre* into a warm bath and enjoy. For gift-giving fill pretty bottles with red or white wine vinegar and add a sprig of dried herb inside the bottle. Red wine vinegar with rosemary is especially festive around the holidays.

Yield: 8 ounces, enough for 1 bath

Rainbow Bath Oil

The age-old saying, "Oil and water don't mix," is the key to this colorful recipe. It's made using two eye-catching colors (I like pink and blue) and can be used as a moisturizing spray, in the bath, or as a light massage oil. If you prefer more natural coloring, choose oils such as extra-virgin olive, avocado, and walnut, which have their own lovely subtle hues.

½ cup light oil (your choice)
½ cup rosewater or orange flower water
2 drops blue food coloring
2 drops red food coloring

Select a clear bottle or container for your oil that has a tight-fitting stopper or lid. Pour the oil into the bottle and add 1–2 drops of the blue food coloring. Shake gently until the oil is lightly colored. In a separate container mix together the rosewater with 1–2 drops of the red food coloring. Pour the colored water into the bottle with the colored oil. The new oil will float to the top.

To use: Shake gently to temporarily mix together the oil and water. The mixture will separate when left to sit, creating a pretty "rainbow" effect. Experiment with other color combinations. The more the oil is shaken, and color is transferred from the oil to the water, the more the color will change.

Yield: 8 ounces

El Dorado Body Oil

¼ cup sesame oil
1 tablespoon wheat germ oil
¼ cup avocado oil
¼ cup almond oil

El Dorado was the name of a South American city of legendary riches sought by Spanish conquistadors. It has become a term used to describe incredible richness—like this recipe rich in natural oils. I think of it as the "El Dorado" of body oils. I like to use it before getting into the shower, since even after washing, it leaves your skin marvelously moisturized. If you wish, you can scent the mixture by adding a few drops of your favorite essential oil or fragrance. I personally prefer it unscented because the natural oils have their own mild scent.

Mix together all the oils and pour into a clean, dry bottle. Shake gently before using.

Yield: 6½ ounces

Disappearing Bath Oil

1 cup light oil (I like to use almond, light sesame, or canola)
½ cup glycerin
½ cup liquid soap

There are two kinds of bath oils: those that float on top of the water (most oils will do this) and those that disperse or disappear into the bathwater. By combining a natural oil together with glycerin and soap, you have a mixture that disperses through your bathwater. You create a bubble bath that works its way beautifully through your bath, leaving your skin soft and smooth. It makes a marvelous gift and can be enhanced by adding your favorite fragrance or scented oil.

Mix together all the ingredients and pour into a clean bottle with a lid or stopper. To use: Shake gently and pour ¼ cup into the bath under running water.

Yield: 16 ounces, enough for 8 baths

Grandfather's Shaving Soap

My grandfather always used a rich shaving soap he kept in a porcelain mug next to his bathroom sink. I used to love watching him shave—painting his face with the thick lather, then removing all traces of soap and beard with a sharp razor. Today, old-style shaving tools are making a comeback as many men are putting down their electric razors for quieter, closer shaves. This shaving soap makes a handsome gift for any well-groomed man on your list. Package it together with a natural-bristle shaving brush or new razor.

¼ cup unscented glycerin soap
½ teaspoon light oil

Melt the soap in the top of a double boiler over boiling water. Blend in the oil. Pour into a clean shaving mug or jar. Let sit until cool and set. To be used with a shaving brush.

Yield: 2 ounces

Tuxedo Cologne

Millionaire Griswold Lorillard caused quite a commotion one night in 1886 when he dared to wear a tailless dress coat to the Tuxedo Club in Tuxedo Park, New York. The new garment was the talk of the nightclub and, of course, was henceforth known as the tuxedo. Today the tuxedo is a must for any properly attired man attending a special affair. Make this impressive cologne and give it to your favorite man before his next big night on the town. This cologne has a fresh, light, spicy scent. And remember: Good grooming is as important as a firm handshake when it comes to making a lasting impression.

½ cup vodka
1 tablespoon champagne
5 black peppercorns
2 dried bay leaves
1 teaspoon grated lime zest
⅛ teaspoon alum powder

Mix together all the ingredients. Pour into a clean jar with a tight-fitting lid. Place the jar in a dark, cool place for 2 weeks, then strain off the liquid and pour into a clean container. Discard any remaining solids. To use: Splash on the face after shaving.

Yield: 4 ounces

Scented Dusting Powder

1 cup cornstarch
1 tablespoon orrisroot powder
1/4 teaspoon essential oil (your choice of scent)

Scented powders absorb and hold fragrance very well. They make wonderful gifts and can be combined in gift baskets with lotions, colognes, and massage oils that have similar scents. Orrisroot powder is used in this recipe as a fixative for the scented oil. It is found in craft shops where potpourri supplies are sold and in natural food stores. Fill a pretty wooden box or decorative tin and include a fluffy powder puff or brush for "dusting" the body.

Place the cornstarch and orrisroot powder in the blender and blend on low speed. With the blender still running, slowly add the essential oil. When well mixed, pour the powder into a clean container.

Yield: 8 ounces

Foaming Bath Salts

½ cup liquid soap
1 tablespoon light oil
Food coloring
6 cups rock salt crystals

These bubbling bath salts are perfect for gift-giving and couldn't be easier to make. They can also be personalized to suit individual tastes. I like to make two batches of this recipe, each one a different color. I then stir the two colors together and pour into large glass jars. You can decorate the jar, embellishing it with glass jewels or silk flowers for a decorative effect.

Mix together the soap, oil, and food coloring. Pour this mixture over the rock salt in a large bowl. Stir continuously until the salt crystals are evenly coated.

Spread the salts out in a thin layer on a cookie sheet covered with wax paper and allow to air-dry. This can take up to 24 hours. Put the bath salts into a decorative container when they are completely dry.

To use: Pour ¼ cup of the salts into the bath under running water.

Yield: 48 ounces, enough for 24 baths

Bath Jelly

½ cup water
1 packet unflavored gelatin
½ cup bubble bath or liquid soap
    (if you're making this for young
    children, use nontoxic,
    nontearing formulas)
Food coloring (optional)
Small plastic toy or seashell

Add this "jelly" to your bathwater for a really invigorating and cleansing experience. Kids especially love this bubbly treat. Create a "Bathtime Basket" to give to your children: Fill a plastic bucket with tubs of bath jelly and include different-shaped sponges, an animal nail brush, bath bubbles (see page 123), and fruit-scented soaps. Make a bath puzzle by cutting up a plastic place mat; when wet, the shapes will stick to the tile walls of your tub or shower.

Heat the water until just boiling and dissolve the gelatin in it. This may take 1–2 minutes.

Add the soap and stir slowly. Do not beat or the soap will become foamy.

Pour the mixture into a plastic container with a lid and drop a small plastic toy or seashell inside as a hidden "surprise."

Place in the refrigerator until set (firm like gelatin). To use: Place a small amount of jelly under the running tap or use as skin cleanser in the tub or shower.

Yield: 8 ounces

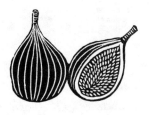

THE PAMPERED BATH BASKET

The bath is the classic setting for pampering oneself. Creating a basket overflowing with bath essentials would be a welcomed bridal shower gift or present for new home (or apartment) owners. It contains everything you need to set up the ultimate bath.

Suggested items to include:

Aphrodite Ocean Bath salts (page 162)

Sea sponges

Foaming Bath Salts (page 225)

Bath brushes

Beautiful Botanical Oils (page 237)

Sensuous Scented Bath Oils (page 58)

Scented candles

Choose a natural basket or wire bath or shower caddie as your container. Line the basket with a fluffy cotton towel or brightly colored rolled-up washcloths. Fill the basket and tie with several strands of raffia. I like to slice off a thin piece of loofah sponge and tie it onto the raffia as a decorative touch to the bow.

Agatha Christie Bath

1 cup fresh apple juice or
    unsweetened bottled apple juice
¼ cup honey
½ cup mild liquid hand or bath
    soap
¼ teaspoon ground cinnamon

My mother loves to read in the bathtub, and one of her favorite authors is the mystery writer Agatha Christie. This seems terribly fitting to me, since Christie herself loved to take long hot baths and eat apples, at the same time! Apples are naturally astringent and contain malic acid, which helps remove dead surface cells, leaving the skin smoother. For a simple present, package this bubble bath with some fresh-picked apples, a good mystery novel, and a new bath pillow.

Stir together all the ingredients and pour into a pretty bottle. To use: Pour ¼–½ cup into the tub under running water. You may need to shake gently to remix ingredients.

Yield: 12 ounces, enough for 3–4 baths

English Mustard Bath

½ cup baking soda
2 tablespoons powdered mustard
2 drops essential oil of peppermint
    (you can also use wintergreen)
2 drops essential oil of rosemary
2 drops essential oil of eucalyptus

In England mustard baths are very popular. They're said to relieve stress, muscle soreness, and sleeplessness caused by anxiety. Mustard is known for its stimulating and cleansing qualities. The warmth of the mustard helps open the pores of your skin, allowing you to sweat out impurities. The scents of peppermint, rosemary, and eucalyptus are all very exciting to the senses. This recipe can be used as a footbath or full body bath. Package this bath powder in an old mustard jar tied up with a checked ribbon and give to an Anglophile friend.

Note: See page 19 on essential oils.

Mix together all ingredients in a glass bowl, stirring until the essential oils are distributed into the powder. To use: Add ¼ cup to the bath under running water.

Relax in the bathtub for 15–20 minutes. After your bath, rinse with a cool shower and pat your skin dry. Dress warmly until your pores are fully closed. For a footbath, add 1 tablespoon of the bath powder to a basin of hot water and then soak your feet for 15 minutes.

Fine Bath Salts

These salts have a finer texture than those made with rock salt, so they will dissolve more quickly. They can also be used as an exfoliating scrub for the body but are too rough for facial use.

Below are listed four different scents for you to concoct. Make one or all four and package them together as a complete set. I like to make pretty paper envelopes and place a small plastic bag with one to two tablespoons of this bath powder inside. They make a sweet little something to tuck into a greeting card or Christmas stocking.

½ cup fine sea salt or table salt
½ cup baking soda
1 teaspoon sunflower oil
2–3 drops essential oils (see suggestions below)
¼ teaspoon vitamin E oil

Place all the ingredients in a resealable plastic bag and knead until well mixed, or you may stir all the ingredients in a glass or ceramic bowl. To use: Add 1–2 tablespoons to your bath under running water.

Yield: 8 ounces, enough for 4 baths

Scents to try:

SWEET ORANGE OIL, LEMON OIL: invigorating and refreshing

LAVENDER OR CHAMOMILE OIL: relaxing and calming

ROSEMARY OIL: stimulating and good for your memory

YLANG-YLANG OR ROSE: uplifting and romantic

BATH TEMPERATURES

The temperature of your bathwater or shower is very important because it can affect your energy level and mood. Take note of the following temperatures and use a thermometer if you have to control the levels. Remember that during the winter, baths that are too hot can really dry out your skin and hair. Never stay in a *very* hot bath for more than fifteen minutes.

Wake-up: A bath or shower set at 70°F–80°F can be very energizing and a great way to start the day.

Warm-up: A short, hot bath or shower set at 102°F can help you warm up if you're chilled, but it is important not to linger more than fifteen minutes at the most.

Fatigue relief: For an instant energizer take a warm bath set at body temperature (98°F–99°F). Soak for about fifteen minutes and you'll feel completely refreshed.

Cool-off: When temperatures outside soar, a bath at just below body temperature, about 92°F, can help you beat the heat. Soak or shower for twenty minutes, and you're guaranteed to feel cool again.

(continued)

Skin-soothing: Adding bath oil to warm water can help soothe dry, itchy skin. Bathwater should be set at 95°F–100°F. Any hotter and it will counteract the oil's moisturizing effect. After bathing, apply more oil to skin while still damp.

Bedtime: If you have trouble sleeping, a short, hot bath before going to bed will help you relax. Water temperature should be above body temperature, 99°F–105°F, but not go over 105°F. Do not bathe or shower for more than fifteen minutes.

Bath Cookies

For those who love to bake, these cookies are fun, fragrant, and nonfattening; in fact, they are good for your skin. They consist of skin-softening sea salt, vitamin E oil, and eggs. Simply drop one or two of these cookie tablets into a warm bath and relax. For gifts I like to package these within colorful tissue paper in decorative tins. Make sure to label them "For the Bath." Although they are basically edible, the large amount of salt makes them undesirable as a tea biscuit!

2 cups finely ground sea salt
½ cup baking soda
½ cup cornstarch
2 tablespoons light oil
1 teaspoon vitamin E oil
2 eggs
5–6 drops essential oil of your
    choice—I like to use chamomile

Preheat your oven to 350°F. Mix together all the ingredients. Take a teaspoon of the dough and roll it gently into a ball (about 1 inch in diameter). Continue doing this with all the dough and place the balls on an ungreased cookie sheet. (You can decorate the cookies with clove buds, anise seeds, or dried citrus peel if you wish.) Bake the cookies for 10 minutes, until they are lightly browned (do not overbake). Allow the cookies to cool completely. To use: Drop 1 or 2 cookies into a warm bath and allow to dissolve.

Yield: 24 cookies, enough for 12 baths

Dill Seed Nail Soak

1 cup boiling water
1 tablespoon dried dill seeds

The dill plant produces a seed that is small, flat, and tan in color. Grown for both the plant and its seeds, dill is a spice that has been used since antiquity in both culinary and cosmetic use. In this recipe the seeds are used to make an excellent nail-strengthening bath. Steeped in boiling water, the seeds produce a liquid that is moisturizing for dry, weak nails. Dill seeds can be found in the spice section of the grocery store or saved from your garden.

Pour the boiling water over the dill seeds and allow them to steep until cool. Strain off the liquid and use as a nail soak or swab onto clean nails nightly.

Yield: 8 ounces

Marathon Massage Oil

One of the largest spectator sports events in the world takes place every November in New York. The New York City Marathon, sponsored by the New York Road Runner's Club, attracts twenty-five thousand participants from all over the world. This recipe makes a welcome gift for your favorite runner or weekend athlete. The camphor in this massage oil is especially soothing to sore, tired muscles. Write a note of encouragement or congratulations and tie around the neck of the bottle—maybe even with the promise of a massage. Package the oil with a large water bottle, some energy bars, and a pair of bright-colored shoelaces, and you have a winning gift.

½ cup light oil (mineral, almond, or safflower)
½ teaspoon camphor oil

Combine the oils and pour into a clean bottle.

Yield: 4 ounces

New-Fashioned Smelling Salts

When I was little, I used to love to go through my grandmother's handbag. She always kept a small bottle of "smelling salts" tucked inside. I never saw her use these salts but suspected they were there just in case she felt "faint." Once I even sniffed the small glass bottle, and I can still remember the strong clear scent of ammonia that filled my head.

Today, I like to keep a small bottle or box of scented salts in my purse or tote bag—not the old-fashioned, ammonia-soaked kind but new-fashioned scented salts to calm my nerves or give me a boost of energy. These small packages make nice gifts individually or in sets of two or three scents, for a variety of moods.

Rock salt
2–3 drops essential oil (see list below for choices)

Fill a small container with the rock salt, then add the chosen essential oil. Keep the lid tightly in place. To use: Smell the salts and try to focus only on the scent; repeat 2 to 3 times.

Calming Scents	Energizing Scents
Basil	Sage
Chamomile	Eucalyptus
Jasmine	Orange
Rose	Lemon
Lavender	Peppermint
Marjoram	Rosemary

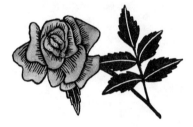

SELF-MASSAGE TOOL

This is a simple massage tool you can make yourself and use for a relaxing back massage. Put two tennis balls, spaced two inches apart, in a clean cotton tube sock. Cut the open end of the sock so it fits around the balls and sew the end of the sock closed. Make a line of stitching on either side of the two-inch space to keep the balls in place. To use: Lie down on your back and position the balls on either side of your backbone. Gently roll up and down, allowing the balls to massage your back.

Simple
Fancy Soaps

If you want to create your own unique gift soaps but don't want to bother with the complete soap-making process (using lye and fat), this is the recipe for you. Using pure soap available at the grocery store, you can make your own unique soap shapes in a variety of colors, scents, and textures—just like those found in many upscale bath shops today. With candy molds, cookie cutters, or other household objects, the possibilities for shapes are endless!

Petroleum jelly for greasing the
   soap molds
1 bar pure white soap (such as
   Ivory or Pure and Natural;
   Castile and glycerin soaps also
   work well), grated—
   approximately 1¼ cups
1 tablespoon water

Note: A simple rule of thumb when melting soap is to use 10 percent of the amount of water to soap. For example, if you have 20 ounces of soap, you would use 2 ounces of water. (An average bar of soap is 3½ to 5 ounces.) I usually use 1 tablespoon (½ ounce) per bar of soap.

Lightly grease the inside of your soap molds using a small amount of petroleum jelly.

Place the soap and water into the top part of a double boiler or in an ovenproof dish in a saucepan of water and heat gently over medium heat. Stir occasionally until all the soap is melted and resembles a smooth, fluffy white pudding. This may take up to 30 minutes. The soap will start out looking very dry and grainy, then turn thick and smooth. Do not allow the mixture to boil.

When all the soap is melted, carefully spoon it into your prepared molds. Overfill the molds just a bit; the soap may settle, and you can always trim away any excess after it has cooled. (You need to work quickly because the soap begins to cool immediately.) Tap the edge of your molds gently to remove any air bubbles.

Allow the molds to sit until the soap is completely cool. Tap the soap shapes from the bottom of the molds and place on a wire baking rack to dry. Let the soap sit for at least 24 hours on the rack. If your shapes seem a bit rough around the edges, you can smooth them out with a sharp knife.

For gift-giving, wrap your soaps in pretty boxes, paper, fabric, or netting tied with ribbon. Do not use airtight containers because it's important to let the soap breathe.

Here are a few variations to try using this basic recipe:

SCENT: If you would like your soap to have a scent, mix in a few drops of your favorite perfumed oil or essential oil after the soap mixture is melted and before you spoon it into your molds. It is important to use oil-based scents because alcohol-based ones may cause your soap to separate.

Soaps also absorb odors, and you can scent your soaps by placing them in a box with petals and leaves from your favorite flowers.

COLOR: You can purchase dyes to use in soap making. I have found simple food coloring, found in the baking section of the grocery store, works quite well. You can also make your own natural dyes using vegetables, herbs, and spices. Green is made using liquid chlorophyll (available at most health food stores). Red can be made from beetroot powder mixed with water or by using strong red herbal teas such as those made with hibiscus flowers. Brown or cream colors can be achieved by using teas such as chamomile and orange pekoe. For yellow you can use saffron or turmeric.

TEXTURE: Another way to add a bit of color and scrubbing power to your soaps is by giving them a texture. Simply add a tablespoon or two of a grainy substance such as cornmeal, ground nuts, or chopped-up loofah sponges to your melted soap before spooning it into the molds. Make sure you stir the mixture thoroughly.

Beautiful Botanical Oils

These beautiful body oils are as pleasing to behold as they are to use. And they're so simple to make. You can literally create dozens of unique combinations in a matter of minutes. It is also an excellent way to use some of the dried herbs and flowers from your summer garden. You may also want to experiment with other natural ingredients placed inside of your bottles: pretty stones, crystals, sea glass, shells, and dried citrus peels knotted or cut into interesting shapes (before drying, of course).

Place dried herbs and flowers into the bottles. When you are pleased with the combinations, fill your bottle with oil, adding a few drops of scent if you wish. The oil will pick up the natural scent from the dried materials over time. Cork or screw on a tight-fitting lid. Label each bottle with the type of oil used and the plant materials it contains.

Small glass bottles, clean and dry
1–2 cups light oil, enough to fill your container (I like to use clear oils such as canola, almond, sunflower and light sesame.)
Assorted dried flowers and herbs (Make sure they are completely dry because moisture will ruin your oil.)
3–4 drops essential oils or scented fragrant oils (optional)

Here are a few of my favorite combinations:

RELAXING: almond oil with dried chamomile flowers, dried yarrow flowers, and dried lavender. Almond oil is slightly yellow in color.

ENERGIZING: avocado oil with dried mint, dried lemon verbena, and dried rosemary. Avocado oil has a slight green tint.

ROMANTIC: mineral oil with dried baby rosebuds, dried lavender flowers, and dried red rose petals. Mineral oil is a very clear oil, and the colors of the flowers become very vibrant.

Note: The longer the oil sits, the stronger its scent will become because it absorbs essential oils and fragrances from the dried flowers and herbs. I like to let my oils sit for at least two weeks before giving them as gifts.

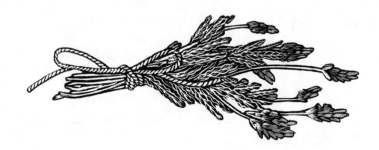

THANKSGIVING BASKET

Thanksgiving is a time for gathering together. For a wonderful hostess gift or a special thank-you this holiday, put together a gift of autumn splendor!

Suggested items to include:

Cranberry Juice Astringent (page 198)

Fresh nuts

Walnut Oil Cream (page 201)

Small pumpkins or gourds

Ginger Hair Oil (page 214)

Marathon Massage Oil (page 233)

Hollow out a large gourd or pumpkin and line it with some natural fabric. Tuck your beauty items inside and place a few sheaves of wheat or a bouquet of dried flowers among the gifts. The dried flowers and wheat can be strewn into warm baths. The fresh nuts, shelled and finely ground, make excellent body scrubs. Use the small pumpkins or gourds (steamed and mashed) to hydrate your skin and hair. Tie several strands of raffia or autumn-colored ribbon around your present. Write a note of thanksgiving and tuck it inside.

Appendix

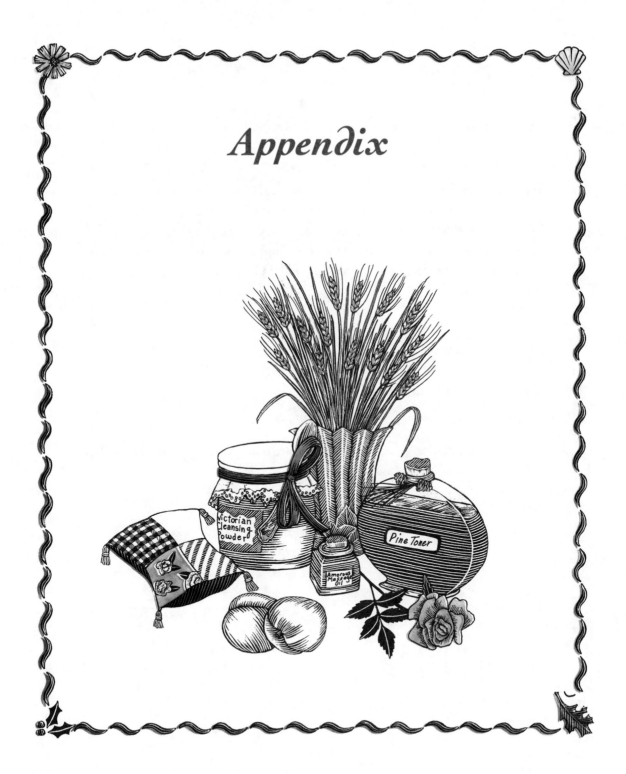

BATH ENVELOPE PATTERN

Trace this pattern onto recycled wrapping paper or plain colored paper, or use a copy machine. Cut out and fold on lines. Glue envelope together and fill with bath salts, powders, herbs, or spices. For recipes that contain oil, I usually place the mixture in a plastic or cellophane bag first and then place the bag inside the envelope. Decorate and label with calligraphy, paint, or stamps.

Assembly Directions:

1. Fold small side flap inward.

2. Spread a small amount of glue along flap.

3. Fold large side flap (envelope back) inward and on top of small side flap. Spread some glue on small bottom flap.

4. Fold up bottom flap on top of envelope back.

5. When glue has dried, fill envelope and fold top flap to close. This flap may be glued in place or held in place with a decorative seal or sticker.

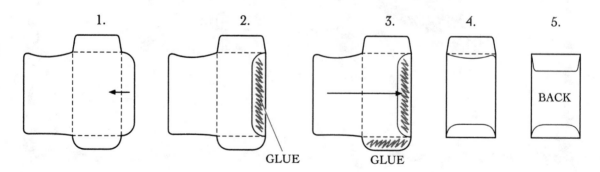

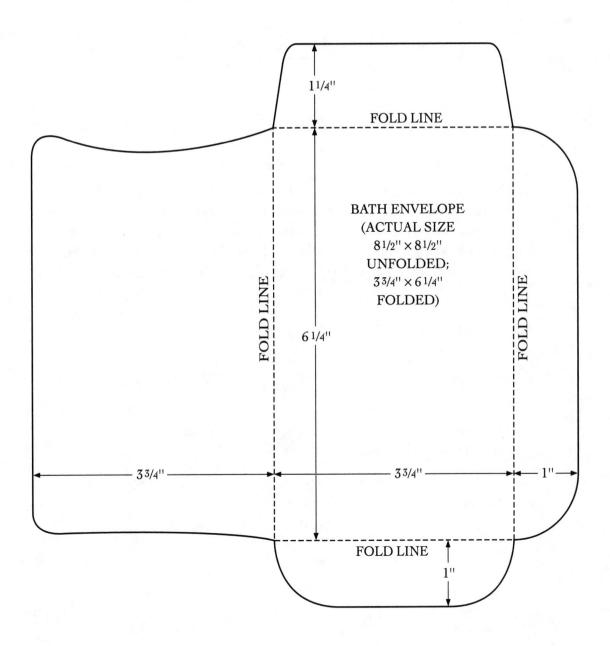

1 1/4"

FOLD LINE

BATH ENVELOPE
(ACTUAL SIZE
8 1/2" × 8 1/2"
UNFOLDED;
3 3/4" × 6 1/4"
FOLDED)

FOLD LINE

FOLD LINE

6 1/4"

3 3/4"

3 3/4"

1"

FOLD LINE

1"

Enlarge at 144% on a photocopier to
create the full-size envelope pattern.

BATH BAG PATTERN

You may purchase small cotton bags—the kind used for sachets and teas—
or create your own from fabric scraps using this pattern. A cotton string or
colorfast ribbon may be used for the drawstrings, and make sure they are
long enough to tie around your tub faucet. Note: If using fabric with a right
side/wrong side, stitch bag with right sides together, then turn right side out.

Assembly Directions:

1. Fold over upper edge along fold line and stitch in place leaving ends
   open.

2. Fold bath bag in half along fold line, right sides together. Stitch ¼-inch
   seam. Turn bag right side out.

3. Thread drawstring through upper casing. (Attach a small safety pin to
   one end of the string to make threading the drawstring much easier and
   remove pin when string is entirely pulled through.)

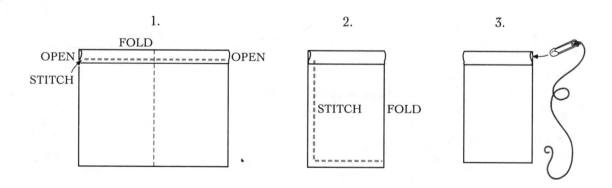

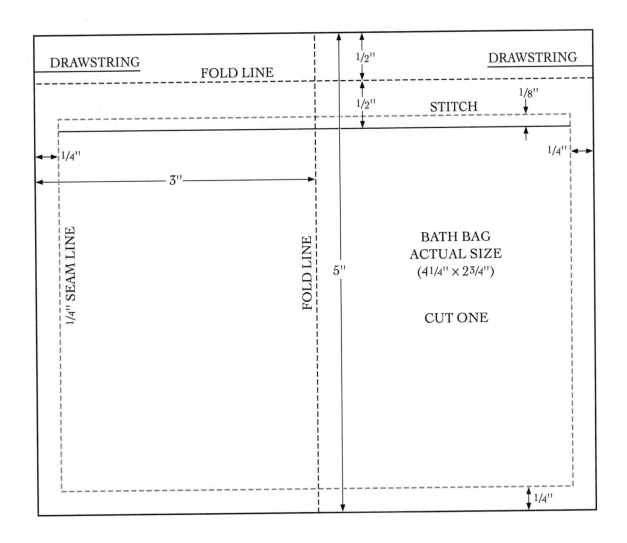

DRAWSTRING   FOLD LINE   DRAWSTRING

1/2"

1/2"

STITCH

1/8"

1/4"

1/4"

3"

FOLD LINE

5"

1/4" SEAM LINE

BATH BAG
ACTUAL SIZE
($4^{1}/4$" × $2^{3}/4$")

CUT ONE

1/4"

FACIAL MASK PATTERN

Use silk or cotton fabric to create a facial mask you can reuse. To use, follow the directions on page 114. Before cutting the material, trace the pattern onto a piece of thin paper and check to see that it fits your face; make changes where needed.

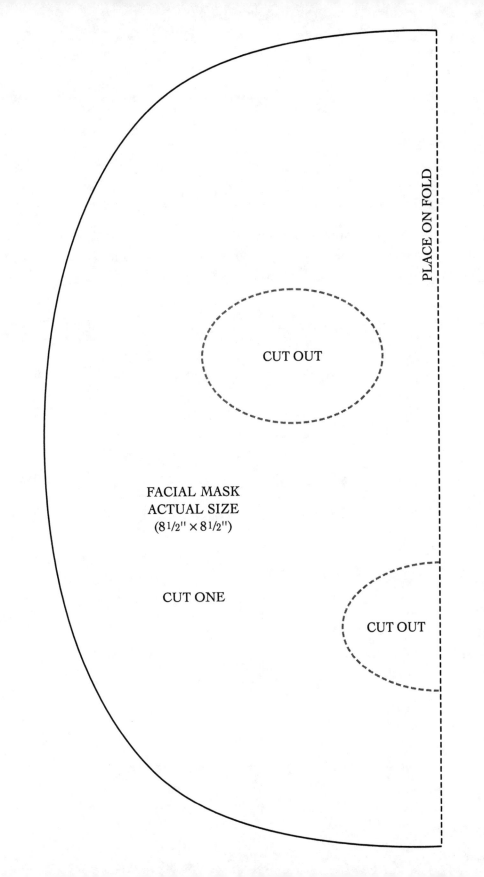

PLACE ON FOLD

CUT OUT

FACIAL MASK
ACTUAL SIZE
($8\frac{1}{2}'' \times 8\frac{1}{2}''$)

CUT ONE

CUT OUT

EYE REST PILLOW PATTERN

You may want to enlarge or shorten this basic pattern. It is designed to fit an average-size face. Follow the directions on page 130 for use and filling instructions.

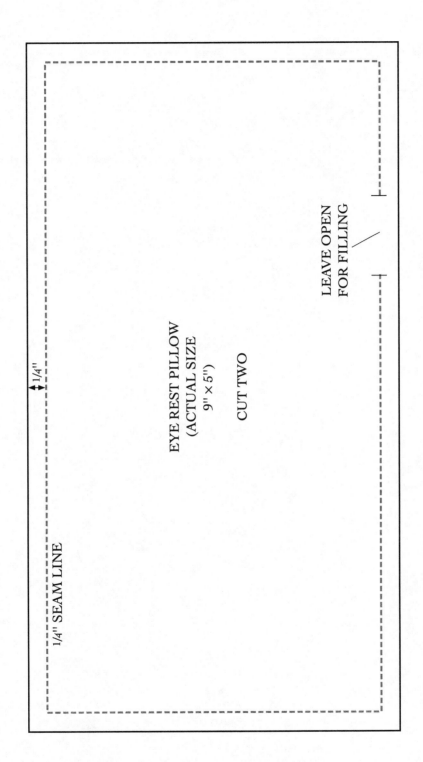

EYE REST PILLOW
(ACTUAL SIZE
9" × 5")

CUT TWO

1/4" SEAM LINE

1/4"

LEAVE OPEN
FOR FILLING

Enlarge at 125% on a photocopier to
create the full-size pillow pattern.

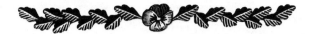

Glossary

Acid: Liquid, solid, or gas that contains hydrogen and reacts with metals to form salts and water. You can usually tell an acid by its pH level, which is below 7. Examples of common acids are citric acid (lemon juice), malic acid (apples), acetic acid (vinegar), and tannic acid (found in tea).

Acid mantle: Microscopic film of acidic moisture over the skin; a kind of protective covering.

Alcohol: Colorless, volatile liquid obtained by distillation and fermentation of carbohydrates (grain, molasses, potatoes). Alcohol is antiseptic and cooling but is also very drying to the hair and skin; care should thus be taken not to use too much.

Anhydrous: Refers to a substance that does not contain water. Lanolin is typically purchased in an anhydrous form.

Antiseptic: A substance that stops the growth of bacteria and helps to control infection by inhibiting germs.

Collagen: The substance that gives skin elasticity, or the ability to stretch. It is found in the inner layer of the skin, or dermis.

Combination skin: Description of skin that has both dry and oily areas. This is the most common skin type.

Cosmetics: Defined by the Federal Drug Act in 1938 (a definition that has not changed) as (1) articles intended to be rubbed, poured, sprinkled, or sprayed on, introduced into, or otherwise applied to the human body or any part thereof for cleansing, beautifying, promoting attractiveness, or altering the appearance, and (2) articles intended for use as a component of any such articles.

Dermis: The inner layer of the skin. The dermis is protected by the epidermis and is made up of tissues, muscles, and nerves. Collagen is found in the dermis layer.

Dry skin: Description of skin that feels tight after washing and has a tendency to flake; the pores are small, and the skin is thin.

Emollient: A thick, creamy material used to soothe or soften the skin. Emollients are usually made from oil, water, and wax. A classic emollient is basic cold cream.

Emulsifier: A material that binds two different materials together. An example of this would be beeswax that is used in making creams to bind together the oil and water and keep them from separating.

Epidermis: The surface layer of the skin. The epidermis is where new cells are constantly being formed.

Exfoliation: Removal of dead skin cells and surface dirt, a very important step in proper skin care because removing dead skin cells allows the skin to function more efficiently and to absorb more moisture.

Facial: A total treatment for the face that consists of deep-cleansing, conditioning, and moisturizing the skin.

Herb: A plant or plant part valued for its medicinal, savory, or aromatic qualities. For example, chamomile is very soothing to the skin, peppermint has a scent that is extremely refreshing, and geranium oil kills bacteria.

Humectant: A substance that holds the moisture in a product or on the skin. Honey is a wonderful natural humectant. Glycerin is the most popular humectant used in cosmetic products.

Infusion: A mixture of herbs and water that has soaked for a period of time. When you make tea, you are making an infusion.

Natural: A term that is loosely used, and no one seems to agree on its definition with regard to cosmetics. The Food and Drug Administration is currently trying to come up with an official definition. I think of natural as not containing any man-made ingredients. Natural to me means "as found in nature." Some feel that natural means no chemicals, but chemicals are natural. Everything in our world is made up of chemical elements.

Normal skin: Clear, firm skin with few blemishes; not dry or oily.

Occlusive oil: A substance that increases the water content of the skin by creating a seal on the surface, holding in moisture. Canola, olive, sesame, and castor oil are all examples of an occlusive oil.

Oily skin: Description of skin that feels a little greasy and has a shine that does not go away, enlarged pores, and no lines.

Organic: A substance that is or once was living. In chemistry, organic means "containing a carbon atom."

pH: The measure of acidity and alkalinity in a solution. The pH scale goes from 0–14 (neutral is 7). Healthy skin may range from pH 3 to 5½.

Ultraviolet light: The invisible rays that penetrate the epidermis and have been proven to cause premature aging and skin cancer.

U.S.P.:   Stands for United States Pharmacopeia and means that the product meets the standards for use set by the United States Pharmaceutical Board. You will see this labeling on many products, such as lanolin, camphor, glycerin, and alum powder.

Water bath: A method for heating ingredients when making cosmetics. A container with ingredients in it is placed in a pan that has one to two inches of water in it. It's similar to a double boiler because it protects ingredients from direct heat. Also known as a *bain marie*. A simple water bath can be made by filling an electric skillet with one to two inches of water.

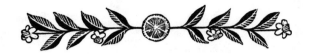

Index